MINDFUL WELLNESS

COPYRIGHT © [2023] BY [JOHNY WRITER]

Mindful wellness is a holistic approach to health that encourages individuals to become aware of their thoughts, feelings and physical sensations in order to develop a sense of self-compassion and inner peace. It is a practice that involves being present in the moment with an open and non-judgmental attitude.

Mindful wellness can be practiced through various techniques such as mindful self-compassion, mindful path to self compassion, mindful therapist, or by using tools such as the mindful way workbook or the healthy mind toolkit. These tools provide guidance on how to create a healthy lifestyle by helping individuals identify their needs and develop healthy habits that are tailored for them. By embracing mindful wellness, individuals can gain insight into their emotions and thoughts in order to better manage stress, anxiety and depression while creating a more balanced life overall. With healthy living made simple and the healthy mind toolkit, you can find the resources you need to take charge of your mental health. This is an opportunity to invest in yourself and take a proactive approach towards improving your physical, mental, emotional, and spiritual wellbeing, healthy progress. Embrace this journey with mindfulness and find out how it can help you lead a more fulfilling life.

A healthy lifestyle is essential for overall well-being and can help prevent a range of health issues, including heart disease, diabetes, and obesity. It involves making healthy choices in your daily life, such as eating a balanced diet, getting enough exercise, and maintaining a healthy weight. It also involves taking care of your mental health, getting enough sleep, and practicing stress management techniques. Maintaining a healthy lifestyle is important for a variety of reasons. For one, it can help you live a longer, healthier life. People who live a healthy lifestyle tend to have lower rates of chronic diseases and conditions, such as heart disease, stroke, diabetes, and cancer. In addition, a healthy lifestyle can improve your mental health and overall quality of life. It can also help you feel more energetic and productive, and can even boost your self-esteem and confidence.

INTRODUCTION:

Living a healthy lifestyle is the key to a happy and productive life. It's not just about eating right and exercising, it's also about having the right tools and information to make informed decisions. That's why we are here to provide you with all the necessary tools and information that you will need to live a healthy lifestyle.

We will cover topics such as nutrition, physical fitness, mental health, stress management, sleep hygiene, relaxation techniques, mindfulness practices, and stress-reducing activities can all be effective ways to reduce stress and improve overall well-being. Relaxation techniques such as deep breathing, progressive muscle relaxation, and yoga can help to calm the mind and body. Mindfulness practices, such as meditation, can help to increase awareness of the present moment and reduce stress by promoting a non-judgmental attitude towards thoughts and feelings. Activities such as exercise, journaling, and spending time in nature can also be effective stress-reducers, as they can help to distract from stressors and promote a sense of calm. Overall, incorporating a variety of relaxation techniques, mindfulness practices, and stress-reducingactivities into your daily routine can help to improve your mental and physical well-being,and more. We will also provide readers with useful tips on how to stay motivated when it comes to living a healthier life.

With our help, you can learn how to make better decisions for your body and mind so that you can be at your best every day!

Chapter 1: Diet and Nutrition

· Discuss the role of nutrition in overall health and well-being.

· Cover the basics of healthy eating, including the importance of a balanced diet, the role of different nutrients, and how to choose nutritious foods.

· Provide tips for meal planning and grocery shopping, including how to read food labels and make healthier choices at restaurants.

Chapter 2: Exercise and Physical Activity

· Explain the benefits of regular physical activity, including improved cardiovascular health, weight management, and stress relief.
· Discuss different types of exercise and the benefits of each, such as strength training, cardiovascular exercise, and flexibility training.
· Offer practical tips for fitting exercise into a busy schedule, including ways to make it enjoyable and rewarding.

Chapter 3: Stress Management

· Discuss the impact of stress on physical and mental health, including the risks of chronic stress.
· Explore different techniques for managing stress, including relaxation techniques, mindfulness practices, and stress-reducing activities.
· Offer tips for identifying and addressing the sources of stress in one's life.

Chapter 4: Sleep and Rest

· Explain the importance of sleep for overall health and well-being.
· Discuss common sleep problems and their causes, as well as strategies for improving sleep quality and quantity.
· Offer tips for creating a sleep-friendly environment and developing healthy sleep habits.

Chapter 5: Personal Care and Self-Care

· Discuss the importance of taking care of oneself, both physically and emotionally.
· Explore different self-care practices, such as skin care, hygiene, and stress-relief techniques.
· Offer tips for developing a self-care routine and making self-care a priority.

CHAPTER 1

HEALTHY EATING

Eating a healthy diet is an important aspect of living a healthy lifestyle. Not only can it help you maintain a healthy weight, it can also reduce your risk of chronic diseases such as heart disease, diabetes, and some types of cancer.

So what does a healthy diet look like? The key is to focus on eating a variety of nutrient-dense foods, rather than just limiting your intake of unhealthy foods. This means choosing whole, unprocessed foods as much as possible and avoiding or minimizing added sugars, salt, and unhealthy fats.

Here are some guidelines for eating a healthy diet:

Include a variety of fruits and vegetables in your diet. Aim for at least 5 servings of fruits and vegetables per day. Choose a variety of colors and types to ensure you are getting a wide range of nutrients.

Choose whole grains over refined grains. Whole grains, such as whole wheat bread, brown rice, and quinoa, are higher in fiber and nutrients than refined grains, such as white bread and pasta.

Include lean protein sources in your diet. Good options include beans, lentils, tofu, poultry, and fish. Avoid or minimize intake of high-fat meats, such as bacon and sausage.

Limit your intake of added sugars and unhealthy fats. This means avoiding sugary drinks and snacks, as well as foods that are high in saturated and trans fats. Instead, choose foods that are rich in healthy fats, such as nuts, seeds, and avocado.

Drink plenty of water. Water is essential for hydration and maintaining proper body function. Aim for at least 8 cups of water per day.

It's also important to pay attention to portion sizes. Even healthy foods can contribute to weight gain if you eat too much of them. Use measuring cups or a food scale to ensure you are getting the right amount of each food group.

Eating a healthy diet can also help improve your mental health and mood. Studies have shown that a diet rich in fruits, vegetables, and other nutrients can help reduce the risk of depression and anxiety. So not only can eating healthy benefit your physical health, it can also benefit your mental well-being.

Of course, it's okay to indulge in your favorite treats every once in a while. The key is to have a healthy balance and not to make unhealthy foods the mainstay of your diet. By following these guidelines and making healthy choices most of the time, you can improve your overall health and well-being.

THE IMPORTANCE OF A BALANCED DIET

A balanced diet is essential for maintaining good health and well-being. It is a diet that includes a variety of different types of foods in the right proportions, providing the body with all the nutrients it needs to function properly.

There are several reasons why a balanced diet is important:

It provides the body with the energy it needs to function properly. Different types of foods provide the body with different types of energy. For example, carbohydrates are a good source of energy for the body, while proteins and fats provide energy at a slower rate.

It helps to maintain a healthy weight. A balanced diet, combined with regular physical activity, can help to maintain a healthy weight. This is important because being overweight or obese can increase the risk of developing chronic health problems such as heart disease, diabetes, and certain types of cancer.

It helps to strengthen the immune system. A balanced diet that is rich in vitamins and minerals can help to boost the immune system, making it more able to fight off infections and illnesses.

It can improve mental health and cognitive function. Some studies have found that a diet that is rich in fruits, vegetables, and other nutrients may help to reduce the risk of depression and improve cognitive function.

It can reduce the risk of chronic diseases. A diet that is balanced and includes a variety of different types of foods may help to reduce the risk of chronic diseases such as heart disease, diabetes, and some types of cancer.

So, what does a balanced diet look like? The key is to include a variety of different types of foods in the right proportions. This means including:

· Fruits and vegetables: Aim for at least 5 servings of fruits and vegetables per day. Choose a variety of colors and types to ensure you are getting a wide range of nutrients.

· Whole grains: Choose whole grains, such as whole wheat bread, brown rice, and quinoa, over refined grains like white bread and pasta.

· Lean protein sources: Good options include beans, lentils, tofu, poultry, and fish. Avoid or minimize intake of high-fat meats like bacon and sausage.

· Healthy fats: Choose foods that are rich in healthy fats, such as nuts, seeds, and avocado, instead of foods high in saturated and trans fats.

· Limited amounts of added sugars and unhealthy fats: Avoid sugary drinks and snacks, as well as foods high in saturated and trans fats.

It's also important to pay attention to portion sizes. Even healthy foods can contribute to weight gain if you eat too much of them. Use measuring cups or a food scale to ensure you are getting the right amount of each food group.

In conclusion, a balanced diet is essential for maintaining good health and well-being. It provides the body with the nutrients it needs to function properly, helps to maintain a healthy weight, strengthens the immune system, and can improve mental health and cognitive function. By including a variety of different types of foods in the right proportions, you can enjoy the many benefits of a balanced diet.

NUTRITIOUS

There are several different types of nutrients that are essential for good health. These nutrients are divided into six main categories: carbohydrates, proteins, fats, vitamins, minerals, and water. Each of these nutrients plays a specific role in the body and is necessary for proper functioning.

Carbohydrates: Carbohydrates are the body's main source of energy. They are found in foods such as grains, fruits, vegetables, and dairy products. There are two main types of carbohydrates: simple and complex. Simple curbs, such as those found in sugary foods and drinks, are quickly absorbed by the body and provide a quick burst of energy. Complex curbs, on the other hand, are found in whole grains, beans, and vegetables and are absorbed more slowly, providing sustained energy.

Proteins: Proteins are essential for the growth, repair, and maintenance of tissues in the body. They are also necessary for the production of enzymes, hormones, and other chemicals. Proteins are made up of smaller units called amino acids. There are 20 different amino acids, and the body needs all of them to function properly. Good sources of protein include meats, beans, nuts, and dairy products.

Fats: Fats are an important source of energy for the body and are necessary for the absorption of certain vitamins and minerals. There are different types of fats, including saturated, monounsaturated, and polyunsaturated fats. Saturated fats, which are found in high-fat meats, full-fat dairy products, and fried foods, should be limited in the diet. Monounsaturated and polyunsaturated fats, which are found in foods such as nuts, seeds, and olive oil, are considered to be more healthful.

Vitamins: Vitamins are essential for the proper functioning of the body's cells, tissues, and organs. They help to regulate many of the body's processes, including the immune system, blood clotting, and metabolism. There are 13 essential vitamins that the body needs, including vitamins A, C, D, E, and K, as well as B vitamins. Good sources of vitamins include fruits, vegetables, and fortified foods.

Minerals: Minerals are essential nutrients that the body needs in small amounts to function properly. They include minerals such as calcium, iron, and zinc. Calcium is necessary for strong bones and teeth, while the iron is essential for the production of red blood cells. Zinc is important for immune function and wound healing. Good sources of minerals include dairy products, meats, and leafy green vegetables.

Water: Water is essential for the proper functioning of the body's cells and organs. It helps to regulate body temperature, transport nutrients, and waste, and lubricate joints. It is important to drink plenty of water to stay hydrated and maintain proper body function.

Nutrients are essential for the proper functioning of the body. They provide the body with energy, help to maintain and repair tissues, and regulate various body processes. By eating a varied diet that includes a variety of different types of nutrients, you can ensure that your body is getting all the nutrients it needs to function properly.

HOW TO CHOOSE NUTRITIOUS FOODS

Eating a healthy diet is an important aspect of living a healthy lifestyle. Choosing nutritious foods is a key part of this process, as it can help you get the nutrients your body needs to function properly and reduce your risk of chronic diseases. However, with so many different types of foods available, it can be difficult to know which ones are the most nutritious. Here are some tips for choosing nutritious foods:

Eat a variety of different types of foods: A diverse diet is more likely to provide you with all the nutrients you need. This means including a variety of different types of fruits and vegetables, whole grains, lean proteins, and healthy fats in your diet.

Choose whole, unprocessed foods: Whole, unprocessed foods are generally more nutritious than processed foods. This is because they are less likely to be stripped of their nutrients during the processing process. Examples of the whole, unprocessed foods include fresh fruits and vegetables, whole grains, and lean proteins.

Look for fortified foods: Some foods are fortified with extra nutrients to make them more nutritious. For example, some types of bread and cereal are fortified with extra vitamins and minerals. Look for these types of fortified foods to boost your nutrient intake.

Read food labels: Food labels can help you make informed decisions about the foods you are eating. Look for foods that are low in added sugars, salt, and unhealthy fats, and high in nutrients such as fiber, protein, vitamins, and minerals.

Choose foods with a lower glycemic index: The glycemic index (GI) is a measure of how quickly a food raises your blood sugar levels. Foods with a high GI are absorbed quickly by the body and can cause a rapid rise in blood sugar, leading to an energy crash. Choose foods with a lower GI, such as whole grains and certain types of fruits and vegetables, to help regulate blood sugar levels and provide sustained energy.

Choose foods with a high nutrient density: Nutrient density refers to the number of nutrients a food provides relative to its calorie content. Foods that are high in nutrients and low in calories are considered to be more nutrient-dense. Examples include leafy green vegetables, berries, and lean proteins.

Don't be afraid to try new foods: Trying new foods can help to expand your palate and increase the variety of nutrients you are getting. Don't be afraid to experiment with different types of fruits, vegetables, and grains to find new foods that you enjoy.

Consider using supplements: While it is generally best to get your nutrients from whole foods, supplements can be a useful addition to your diet in certain situations. For example, if you have a specific nutrient deficiency or are at risk of a deficiency due to a medical condition, a supplement may be necessary to help fill the nutrient gap. However, it is important to talk to a healthcare provider before starting any new supplements, as they can interact with certain medications and have potential side effects.

By choosing nutritious foods is an important aspect of maintaining good health and well-being. By eating a diverse diet that includes a variety of different types of whole, unprocessed foods, and by reading food labels and looking for fortified foods, you can ensure that you are getting all the nutrients your body needs to function properly. Don't be afraid to try new foods and consider using supplements in certain situations, but always talk to a healthcare provider before starting any new supplements.

Meal planning and grocery shopping: Are important tasks that can help you eat a healthy diet and save time and money. By planning your meals in advance and making a shopping list, you can ensure that you have the ingredients you need to make healthy meals and snacks. Here are some tips for meal planning and grocery shopping:

Start by making a list of your favorite healthy meals and snacks: Consider what types of foods you enjoy eating and how they fit into a healthy diet. This can help you come up with ideas for meals and snacks that you will look forward to eating.

Plan your meals and snacks for the week: Once you have a list of your favorite healthy meals and snacks, start planning out what you will eat for each meal and snack for the week. Consider any commitments you have, such as work or school, and plan accordingly.

Make a grocery list: Based on your meal plan, make a list of the ingredients you will need for the week. This will help you stay organized and ensure that you don't forget any important items.

Shop with a budget in mind: Determine how much money you have available for groceries and try to stick to this budget as closely as possible. Look for sales and discounts, and consider purchasing store brands to save money.

Shop the perimeter of the store first: The perimeter of the store is usually where the fresh produce, meats, and dairy products are located. By shopping these areas first, you can focus on purchasing healthy, whole foods.

Don't shop when you are hungry: It can be tempting to purchase unhealthy snacks or foods when you are hungry, so try to shop on a full stomach to avoid this temptation.

Consider purchasing frozen or canned produce: Frozen and canned produce can be a convenient and cost-effective option, especially if you can't find fresh produce that is in season. Just be sure to check the label for added sugars, salts, and preservatives.

Consider purchasing bulk items: Buying in bulk can be a cost-effective option, especially for items that you use frequently, such as grains, nuts, and seeds. Just be sure to store these items properly to prevent spoilage.

Don't be afraid to try new foods: Trying new foods can help to expand your palate and increase the variety of nutrients you are getting. Don't be afraid to experiment with different types of fruits, vegetables, and grains to find new foods that you enjoy.

Consider using meal delivery or meal prep services: If you don't have the time or energy to meal plan and grocery shop, consider using a meal delivery or meal prep service. These services can provide you with pre-made or pre-packaged meals and snacks, saving you time and effort.

Meal planning and grocery shopping are important tasks that can help you eat a healthy diet and save time and money. By making a list of your favorite healthy meals and snacks, planning your meals and snacks for the week, and making a grocery list, you can stay organized and ensure that you have the ingredients you need to make healthy meals and snacks. Consider shopping the perimeter of the store, purchasing frozen or canned produce, and using meal delivery or meal prep services to make the process easier. Don't be afraid to try new foods and shop with a budget in mind to save money.

Reading food labels: Is an important skill that can help you make informed decisions about the foods you are eating. Food labels provide important information about the nutrients, ingredients, and serving sizes of food, and can help you choose healthier options. Here are some tips for reading food labels:

Look at the serving size: The serving size listed on the food label is the amount of the food that is considered to be a single serving. This is important to pay attention to, as the nutrient content listed on the label is based on this serving size. If you eat more or less than the serving size listed, you will need to adjust the nutrient content accordingly.

Check the calorie content: The calorie content listed on the food label is the amount of energy the food provides. If you are trying to lose weight, you may want to choose foods that are lower in calories. However, it's important to note that not all calories are created equal, and some foods that are high in calories may also be high in nutrients.

Check the fat content: The fat content listed on the food label includes the total amount of fat in the food, as well as the amount of saturated and trans fats. Saturated and trans fats are considered to be less healthful than unsaturated fats and should be limited in the diet. Choose foods that are low in saturated and trans fats and high in unsaturated fats, such as nuts and seeds.

Check the carbohydrate content: The carbohydrate content listed on the food label includes the total amount of carbohydrates in the food, as well as the amount of fiber and sugar. Choose foods that are high in fiber and low in added sugars, as these types of carbohydrates are generally more healthful.

Check the protein content: The protein content listed on the food label is the amount of protein in the food. Protein is an important nutrient that is necessary for the growth, repair, and maintenance of tissues in the body.
Choose foods that are high in protein, such as lean meats, beans, and nuts.

Check the ingredient list: The ingredient list on the food label lists all of the ingredients in the food, in descending order by weight. Look for whole, unprocessed ingredients and avoid foods that contain a lot of added sugars, salts, and unhealthy fats.

Look for fortified foods: Some foods are fortified with extra nutrients to make them more nutritious. For example, some types of bread and cereal are fortified with extra vitamins and minerals. Look for these types of fortified foods to boost your nutrient intake.

Check the expiration date: The expiration date on the food label indicates when the food is no longer safe to eat. Make sure to check the expiration date before purchasing food to ensure that it is still fresh.

Consider the serving size when comparing foods: When comparing different types of foods, it's important to consider the serving size. For example, if one food has more calories or fat per serving than another, but the serving size is smaller, it may still be a healthier option.

Reading food labels is an important skill that can help you make informed decisions about the foods you are eating.

Eating out at restaurants can be a convenient and enjoyable way to try new foods and socialize with friends and family. However, it can also be a challenge to make healthy choices when dining out, as many restaurant meals are high in calories, fat, and sodium. Here are some tips for making healthier choices at restaurants:

Look for healthy options on the menu: Many restaurants now offer healthier options on their menus, such as salads, grilled chicken or fish, and steamed vegetables. Look for these types of options, as they are generally lower in calories and fat than fried or creamy dishes.

Ask for modifications to your meal: If you don't see any healthy options on the menu that appeal to you, consider asking the server if they can make modifications to a dish to make it healthier. For example, you could ask for grilled chicken instead of fried, or request that sauce or dressing be served on the side so you can control the amount you use.

Share a dish with a friend: Many restaurant portions are larger than the recommended serving size, so consider sharing a dish with a friend or family member to reduce the number of calories you are consuming. Order vegetables as an accompaniment to a meal. Consider ordering one of these options as an additional source of nutrients.

Choose water or unsweetened drinks: Sugary drinks, such as soda and sweetened coffee and tea, can add a lot of calories to a meal. Choose water or unsweetened drinks instead to save calories and sugar.

Don't be afraid to ask questions: If you have any questions about the ingredients or preparation of a dish, don't be afraid to ask the server or chef. They may be able to provide you with more information about the meal and help you make a healthier choice.

Look for nutrition information: Some restaurants now provide nutrition information on their menus or online. This can be a helpful resource for making healthier choices.

Consider the type of restaurant: Different types of restaurants may have different types of healthier options available. For example, a salad bar or a health-focused restaurant may have more options that fit into a healthy diet.

Plan ahead: If you know you will be eating out at a restaurant, consider making healthier choices earlier in the day to balance out.

Eating a healthy diet is an important aspect of maintaining good health and well-being. A healthy diet includes a variety of different types of nutritious foods that provide the body with the energy and nutrients it needs to function properly.

One key aspect of a healthy diet is balance. A balanced diet includes a variety of different types of nutrients, including carbohydrates, proteins, fats, vitamins, minerals, and water. Each of these nutrients plays a specific role in the body and is necessary for proper functioning. By eating a varied diet that includes a variety of different types of nutrients, you can ensure that your body is getting all the nutrients it needs to function properly.
To choose nutritious foods, it is important to focus on whole, unprocessed foods that are high in nutrients and low in added sugars, salts, and unhealthy fats. You can also look for fortified foods that are enriched with extra nutrients, and read food labels to make informed decisions about the foods you are eating.

Meal planning and grocery shopping are important tasks that can help you eat a healthy diet and save time and money. By making a list of your favorite healthy meals and snacks, planning your meals and snacks for the week, and making a grocery list, you can stay organized and ensure that you have the ingredients you need to make healthy meals and snacks. Consider shopping the perimeter of the store, purchasing frozen or canned produce, and using meal delivery or meal prep services to make the process easier. Don't be afraid to try new foods and shop with a budget in mind to save money.

When dining out at restaurants, it can be a challenge to make healthy choices. To make healthier choices at restaurants, look for healthy options on the menu, ask for modifications to your meal, share a dish with a friend, order a side salad or vegetables, choose water or unsweetened drinks, and consider the type of restaurant. You can also look for nutrition information and don't be afraid to ask questions about the ingredients or preparation of a dish. By making these healthier choices, you can enjoy dining out while still maintaining a healthy diet.

CHAPTER 2

Regular physical activity: Is an important aspect of maintaining good health and well-being. It can help to improve cardiovascular health, increase strength and flexibility, and reduce the risk of chronic diseases such as obesity, type 2 diabetes, and heart disease. Here are some specific benefits of regular physical activity:

Weight management: Physical activity can help to maintain a healthy weight by burning calories and increasing muscle mass. This can be especially important for people who are trying to lose weight or prevent weight gain.

Improved cardiovascular health: Regular physical activity can help to improve cardiovascular health by increasing heart and lung function, lowering blood pressure, and improving blood cholesterol levels. This can reduce the risk of heart disease and stroke.

Increased strength and flexibility: Physical activity can help to build and maintain muscle strength and flexibility, which can improve balance and coordination and reduce the risk of falls and injuries.

Improved mental health: Physical activity has been shown to improve mood, reduce stress and anxiety, and improve sleep quality. It can also help to increase self-esteem and self-confidence.

Increased bone density: Regular physical activity can help to increase bone density and reduce the risk of osteoporosis, a condition that causes the bones to become weak and brittle.

Improved cognitive function: Physical activity has been shown to improve cognitive function, including memory and problem-solving skills. It can also help to reduce the risk of cognitive decline and dementia.

Increased lifespan: Studies have shown that regular physical activity can increase lifespan and reduce the risk of premature death from chronic diseases.

Improved quality of life: Physical activity can improve overall quality of life by increasing energy levels, improving sleep, and reducing the risk of chronic diseases.

Regular physical activity is an important aspect of maintaining good health and well-being. It can help to improve cardiovascular health, increase strength and flexibility, and reduce the risk of chronic diseases. It can also improve mental health, increase bone density, improve cognitive function, increase lifespan, and improve the overall quality of life. By incorporating regular physical activity into your lifestyle, you can enjoy these many benefits and improve your overall health and well-being.

Weight management is an important factor to consider when it comes to maintaining a healthy lifestyle. Excess weight can lead to an increased risk of developing chronic diseases and can also contribute to a decrease in overall quality of life. It is important to maintain a healthy weight by engaging in regular physical activity and following a nutritious diet. By doing so, you can reduce your risk of developing chronic diseases, enjoy an improved quality of life, and potentially increase your lifespan.

Along with regular physical activity, it is important to maintain a healthy weight. Weight management is key to leading a healthy lifestyle, as it can help reduce the risk of chronic diseases, such as heart disease and type 2 diabetes. Eating a balanced diet and getting enough sleep can also contribute to weight management and help you maintain a healthy lifestyle. Additionally, regular physical activity can help you reach and maintain a healthy weight, allowing you to experience the many benefits of living a healthy lifestyle.

Weight management is an important aspect of maintaining good health and well-being. Having a healthy weight can help to reduce the risk of chronic diseases, such as obesity, type 2 diabetes, and heart disease, and can improve the overall quality of life. Here are some specific ways in which weight management is important for healthy living:

Reducing the risk of chronic diseases: Being overweight or obese is a major risk factor for chronic diseases such as type 2 diabetes, heart disease, and certain types of cancer. By maintaining a healthy weight, you can reduce your risk of these diseases and improve your overall health.

Improving physical health: Maintaining a healthy weight can help to improve physical health in a number of ways. It can help to reduce joint strain and lower the risk of osteoarthritis, improve cardiovascular health, and increase energy levels.

Improving mental health: Weight management can also have a positive impact on mental health. Being overweight or obese has been linked to an increased risk of depression and anxiety, and losing weight can help to improve self-esteem and body image.

Increasing lifespan: Studies have shown that people who are overweight or obese have a higher risk of premature death compared to those who are at a healthy weight. By maintaining a healthy weight, you can increase your lifespan and enjoy a higher quality of life.

Reducing healthcare costs: Maintaining a healthy weight can also help to reduce healthcare costs. Chronic diseases such as obesity and type 2 diabetes can be expensive to treat, and by maintaining a healthy weight, you can reduce your risk of these diseases and lower your healthcare costs.

To maintain a healthy weight, it is important to engage in regular physical activity and eat a healthy diet. Aim for at least 150 minutes of moderate-intensity activity or 75 minutes of vigorous-intensity activity per week, or a combination of both. Choose a variety of whole, unprocessed foods that are high in nutrients and low in added sugars, salts, and unhealthy fats, and avoid overeating. It may also be helpful to track your food intake and physical activity using a food diary or Smartphone app and to seek support from friends, family, or a healthcare professional if you need help with weight management.

Weight management: Is an important aspect of maintaining good health and well-being. By maintaining a healthy weight, you can reduce your risk of chronic diseases, improve physical and mental health, increase lifespan, and reduce healthcare costs. By engaging in regular physical activity and eating a healthy diet, you can achieve and maintain a healthy weight and enjoy a healthier lifestyle.

Stress is a normal part of life, and can be caused by a variety of factors such as work, family, relationships, and daily responsibilities. While some stress can be helpful in motivating us to meet deadlines or perform at our best, chronic stress can have negative effects on our physical and mental health. Here are some reasons why stress relief is important:

Reducing the risk of physical health problems: Chronic stress has been linked to a number of physical health problems, such as heart disease, high blood pressure, and weakened immune function. By finding ways to reduce stress, you can reduce your risk of these health problems and improve your overall physical health.

Improving mental health: Stress can also have negative effects on mental health, such as causing anxiety, depression, and sleep problems. By finding ways to relieve stress, you can improve your mental health and well-being.

Increasing productivity: Chronic stress can interfere with productivity and concentration, making it more difficult to get things done. By finding ways to relieve stress, you can improve your focus and productivity.

Improving relationships: Stress can also have negative effects on relationships, as it can cause conflicts and misunderstandings. By finding ways to relieve stress, you can improve communication and strengthen your relationships.

There are many different ways to relieve stress, including exercise, relaxation techniques, such as deep breathing and meditation, and hobbies or activities that you enjoy. It may also be helpful to talk to a healthcare professional or a counselor if you are experiencing chronic stress and are having difficulty managing it on your own.

Stress relief is important for maintaining good physical and mental health and well-being. By finding ways to relieve stress, you can reduce your risk of physical health problems, improve your mental health, increase productivity, and improve your relationships. Finding effective stress relief strategies can be challenging, as different methods may work better for different people. However, it is important to experiment and to find what works for you. There are many different ways to relieve stress, and it may be helpful to try a variety of techniques to find what works best for you. From physical activities to mindfulness exercises, there are plenty of strategies that can help you manage stress and lead a healthier, happier life.

There are different types of exercise and the benefits of each, such as strength training, cardiovascular exercise, and flexibility training.

Exercise: Is an important part of stress management. Different types of exercise offer different benefits, and it may be helpful to experiment with different activities to find what works best for you. Strength training helps build muscle, cardiovascular exercise helps improve your overall cardiovascular health, and flexibility training helps increase the range of motion in your joints. Incorporating a variety of exercises can also help keep you motivated and engaged in your routine.

There are many different types of exercise that can help to reduce stress and improve overall physical and mental health. Strength training exercises can help to increase muscle mass, improve physical fitness, and reduce stress. Cardiovascular exercises, such as running, cycling, and swimming, can help to improve heart health, lower blood pressure, and reduce stress. Finally, flexibility training exercises, such as stretching, yoga, and Pilates, can help to improve the range of motion, reduce stiffness, and improve overall well-being.

Exercise is an important aspect of maintaining good health and well-being, but it can be challenging to fit it into a busy schedule. Here are some practical tips for fitting exercise into a busy schedule:

Make a plan: Set specific times for exercise each week and schedule them into your calendar as you would any other important commitment. Consider finding a workout buddy or joining a class to help hold yourself accountable.

Find an activity you enjoy: Choose an exercise activity that you enjoy, whether it's a sport, a group fitness class, or a solo activity like running or yoga. You are more likely to stick with an activity if it is something you enjoy.

Keep it short and simple: If you don't have a lot of time, try to fit in short, intense workouts that can be done in just a few minutes. Bodyweight exercises, such as push-ups, squats, and lunges, can be done anywhere and don't require any equipment.

Make it a habit: Incorporate physical activity into your daily routine by taking the stairs instead of the elevator, walking or biking to work, or going for a walk during your lunch break.

Find a workout buddy: Working out with a friend can be a great way to stay motivated and have fun. It can also help to hold you accountable and make the time go by faster.

Reward yourself: Celebrate your progress and reward yourself for reaching your fitness goals. This could be something as simple as treating yourself to a new workout outfit or a healthy meal.

Be flexible: It's okay if you can't fit in a long workout every day. Even short bursts of physical activity, such as a 10-minute walk, can have health benefits. The important thing is to be consistent and make exercise a regular part of your routine.

Fitting exercise into a busy schedule can be challenging, but it is possible with a little planning and dedication. By finding an activity you enjoy, keeping it short and simple, and making it a habit, you can make exercise an enjoyable and rewarding part of your daily routine.

CHAPTER 3

Stressis a normal and natural part of life, and everyone experiences stress to some degree. Stress can be caused by a variety of factors, such as work, relationships, or financial concerns, and can be either positive or negative. Positive stress, also known as esters, can motivate and energize us, while negative stress, also known as distress, can be harmful to our health.

The impact of stress on physical and mental health can vary depending on the severity and duration of the stress. Chronic stress, which is prolonged and ongoing stress, can have particularly negative impacts on health. Chronic stress can weaken the immune system, increase the risk of heart disease and stroke, and contribute to the development of mental health disorders such as depression and anxiety.

Here are some specific ways in which stress can impact physical and mental health:

Physical health

Stress can have a number of negative impacts on physical health. It can weaken the immune system, making it more difficult to fight off infections and diseases. Chronic stress has also been linked to an increased risk of heart disease and stroke, as well as digestive problems, headaches, and sleep disturbances.

Mental health

Stress can also have negative impacts on mental health. It can contribute to the development of mental health disorders such as depression and anxiety, and can also worsen symptoms of these conditions. Stress can also interfere with memory and concentration and can lead to feelings of irritability, anger, and hopelessness.

Behavior

Stress can affect behavior in a number of ways. It can lead to unhealthy behaviors such as overeating, smoking, or excessive alcohol consumption, which can further contribute to physical and mental health problems. Stress can also cause people to become more isolated and withdraw from social activities, which can further contribute to feelings of loneliness and isolation.

To manage stress and reduce its negative impacts on health, it is important to find effective coping mechanisms. Some effective stress management techniques include exercise, relaxation techniques, time management, supportive relationships, and healthy lifestyle habits. By finding ways to manage stress and reduce its negative impacts on health, you can improve your physical and mental well-being and enjoy a better quality of life.

There are many different techniques that can be used to manage stress and reduce its negative impacts on health. Here are some effective stress management techniques:

Exercise

Regular physical activity can help to reduce stress by releasing endorphins, which are chemicals that improve mood and reduce feelings of stress. Exercise can also help to reduce tension and improve sleep quality, which can further help to reduce stress.

Relaxation techniques

Relaxation techniques such as deep breathing, meditation, or progressive muscle relaxation can help to calm the mind and reduce stress. These techniques can be practiced anywhere and can be especially useful when you are feeling overwhelmed or anxious.

Time management

Managing time effectively can help to reduce stress by ensuring that tasks are completed on time and that you have time for relaxation and leisure activities. This can be achieved through techniques such as setting goals, prioritizing tasks, and delegating responsibilities.

Supportive relationships

Having a strong support system of friends and family can help to reduce stress by providing a sense of belonging and connection. It can also be helpful to seek support from a mental health professional if you are experiencing chronic or severe stress.

HEALTHY LIFESTYLE HABITS

Maintaining a healthy diet, getting enough sleep, and engaging in regular physical activity can all help to reduce stress and improve overall health. It is also important to avoid unhealthy behaviors such as overeating, smoking, or excessive alcohol consumption, which can further contribute to stress and other health problems.

Coping skills

Developing coping skills such as problem-solving, communication, and assertiveness can help you to better manage stress and handle difficult situations. It can also be helpful to learn to accept things that you cannot change and to identify and change negative thinking patterns.

Hobbies and leisure activities

Engaging in hobbies and leisure activities that you enjoy can help to reduce stress by providing a sense of accomplishment and a break from daily responsibilities. These activities can also provide a sense of connection to others and a sense of purpose.

Relaxation

Relaxation techniques are a type of stress management technique that can help to calm the mind and reduce stress. These techniques work by focusing the mind on a specific task or activity, which helps to divert attention away from stressors and promotes a state of relaxation. Relaxation techniques can be practiced anywhere and can be especially useful when you are feeling overwhelmed or anxious. Here are some common relaxation techniques are:

Deep breathing

Deep breathing involves taking slow, deep breaths in through the nose and exhaling slowly through the mouth. This technique can help to relax the muscles and calm the mind. It is especially helpful when used in combination with other relaxation techniques, such as progressive muscle relaxation.

MEDITATION

Meditation involves focusing the mind on a specific object, thought, or activity, and letting go of all other thoughts. This can be achieved through techniques such as mindfulness meditation, in which you focus on the present moment, or visualization, in which you create a peaceful mental image. Meditation can help to reduce stress and improve focus and concentration.

If you're just starting started with meditation, I recommend keeping things easy. Here are a few pointers:

Find a comfortable sitting position for yourself. It is OK to use a chair or a cushion on the floor, whatever is more comfortable for you. It is also OK to be slightly reclined as long as your spine, neck, and head are all in a straight line. It is beneficial to have a certain meditation area and chair or cushion that you utilize whenever possible (although it is also fine to meditate wherever you are if the spirit moves you). If you choose, you can adorn that area of your home with flowers, candles, or other spiritual artifacts.
The easiest thing to concentrate on is your own breath. You can just observe the sensations of your air entering and exiting your nostrils. When your mind wanders, gently bring it back to the breath. It is totally normal for the mind to stray; just keep bringing it back to the breath. You don't need to adjust your breathing pattern or breathe more deeply. Simply observe the feelings in your nose while you breathe normally.

It is beneficial to remain as physically motionless as possible throughout the meditation, as well as to keep your eyes behind your closed eyelids steady. Simply let your eyes fall into their sockets and remain still.

Begin with whatever amount of time is comfortable for you and progressively increase the amount of time you sit. You may notice that lengthier meditations have different results, but allow yourself to gradually increase the duration every week or so to enable your body and mind to acclimatize and create a consistent habit without becoming overwhelmed or disappointed. Recent neuroscience research has indicated that extended meditation sessions lasting an hour or more are far more beneficial. This may seem like a lot to a beginner, but after you experience the more powerful benefits of longer meditations, you may find yourself wanting to meditate for larger periods of time. I would definitely recommend practicing one lengthy meditation each day rather than two shorter meditations. Initially, I found it beneficial to meditate first thing in the morning and/or the last thing at night. This is a simple method to incorporate into your daily routine since there is always more time at the start and end of the day if you just wake up earlier or go to bed a bit later.

The only way to tell whether you had a "good" meditation is if you stayed on the chair/cushion the entire time. Meditation works by repetition, so even if your mind wanders or you believe nothing is happening, if you are still sitting on your cushion when the timer goes off, it was a "good" meditation.
If you want to incorporate a basic breathing method, I recommend performing alternate nostril breathing for 10 minutes or so before you meditate, and then simply following your breath throughout your meditation.

PROGRESSIVE MUSCLE RELAXATION

Progressive muscle relaxation involves tensing and relaxing different muscle groups in a specific order. This technique can help to reduce muscle tension and promote relaxation. To practice progressive muscle relaxation, start by tensing a muscle group for a few seconds, then relaxing it for a few seconds before moving on to the next muscle group.

Guided imagery

Guided imagery involves creating a peaceful mental image and focusing on it in order to relax the mind and body. This technique can be practiced with the help of a recorded script or with the guidance of a trained therapist.

YOGA

Yoga involves a series of physical postures, breathing techniques, and meditation practices that can help to promote relaxation and reduce stress. Yoga can also improve flexibility and strength and has been shown to have a number of other health benefits.

Establish a cozy space for your yoga practice.
It's excellent if you have a spare room you can use for yoga. It is undoubtedly enticing to keep your yoga mat unrolled and available at all times.

However, the majority of us must be more adaptable and make a place where we wish to practice. Find a place with as much open space as you can, where it's calm and pleasant. Given how useful the wall is as a prop, an empty section of it can also come in handy. If you like, lighting a candle or an incense stick might help set the mood and be lovely.

Candles and incense are optional and not at all required to practice yoga; they are just nice to have. As long as there is enough room around you without the fear of running into tables, chairs, etc., you may practice yoga anyplace. I've practiced in the living room while my spouse reads the newspaper and eats breakfast, occasionally adding a comment. Although not ideal, I still managed to practice, which is the article's main takeaway.
Therefore, think beyond the box and stretch out on your mat. Make the best practice area you can, and have fun!

Obtain yoga equipment.

Really, all you need is a yoga mat—preferably one that won't slip." Despite the big yoga mat market, it's worthwhile to spend a little extra money on a high-quality mat that will meet your demands and endure for a very long time. Blocks are a terrific addition, but you may also use books and other household items in their place.

Although having a bolster is lovely, for years I substituted a stack of pillows and blankets.

No equipment, not even a yoga mat, is necessary to practice. Accessories and even a yoga mat are not necessary to practice; in locations where there was no yoga mat, I was able to use a piece of carpet. Even in hotel rooms when there wasn't enough to spread out a mat, I've practiced on mattresses. Simply be inventive; make no excuses.

Remain secure and avoid harm

There are no quick cuts for this advice. Always be aware of your boundaries, and pay particular attention to the weak points in your body. The neck, spine, and knees are particularly delicate regions. If you experience any discomfort, make any adjustments, soften, or exit the posture. Don't push or use force.

Before attempting more difficult positions, thoroughly warm up your body. While in a pose, continuously check to see whether it feels comfortable. Take extra care while entering or exiting positions or changing poses because these are times when we tend to pay less attention to our alignment which might result in injury.

Select your yoga schedule or style

When you are on your mat, what will you do? The first thing to consider is what your body and mind require.

Something energizing like Vinnitsa Flow, or something gentler and restorative, to calm your body and mind? The more yoga you practice, the more you become aware of the impact of various techniques and the diverse needs your body and mind may have at various times.

Avoid spending too much time reading class descriptions if you decide to take an online course. The human mind is wired to seek the ideal category to account for every problem. You have to create that class yourself because it doesn't exist. You may also select from one of our yoga programs, which are collections of courses that go well together, or from one of our Playlists, which are collections of classes created by Yoga teachers and other members of the community.

Choose a style, teacher, particular usage, and ideal class length (or any combination of these) from the filters on the courses page, then go for it! With as little resistance as possible, you may practice in a style that makes the lesson ideal for you. Breathe through any parts you find objectionable while keeping an eye on your emotions. Keep in mind that your daily behavior is influenced by how you behave on the mat. You will also encounter situations in daily life that you don't like but can't or won't alter. Keep in mind the advice of Pattabhi Jois: "Do your practice and all will come."

You will learn to submit to what is when you practice yoga on your mat over time. You'll discover how to stop battling the status quo and giving up on making changes. After that, you'll be able to use that outlook more in your life off the mat. I guarantee you'll enjoy the tranquility that comes with being able to accept the way things are.

Your yoga mat practice will gradually educate you to give more and more of yourself up to the world as it is. You'll discover how to give up attempting to alter things and giving up opposing what is. Then, you'll be better able to use that outlook in your life off the mat. I assure you that the tranquility that comes from being able to accept what is tremendous.

Constantly unwind with Savasana

Giving your body enough time to unwind in Savasana after a yoga session is crucial. The advantages of the exercise must be assimilated by the neurological system over time. Otherwise, especially after a hard yoga session, you could feel overly wired after your yoga practice.

Regularly practice yoga

Yoga is healthy, even only once a week! Both three times each week and every day are excellent. What operates for you? If achieving objectives is really important to you, setting a goal of practicing three times per week, being able to do it, and feeling pleased with yourself is preferable to set a goal of practicing every day and feeling horrible if you only manage it three times per week. You often miss practices much more when you feel unsuccessful. As a result, be truthful, make sensible goals, and take action. Yoga poses performed for 10 minutes still qualify as practice.

Mindfulness

Mindfulness is the energy that allows us to perceive the joyful conditions that are already present in our life. You don't have to wait ten years to find happiness. It is there at all times in your daily life. There are those of us who are alive but are unaware of it. However, as you breathe in and become aware of your in-breath, you experience the marvel of being alive. That is why mindfulness brings happiness and joy. The majority of individuals are forgetful; they are not always there. Their thoughts are caught up in their worries, anxieties, wrath, and regrets, and they are unaware that they are there. That is referred to as forgetfulness—you are present but not present. You're stuck in the past or the future. You are not there in the moment, enjoying your life fully. That is the definition of forgetting.

Mindfulness is the polar opposite of forgetting. Mindfulness is when your mind and body are genuinely present. You take attentive breaths in and out, return your attention to your body, and you are there. When your mind and body are in sync, you are in the present moment. Then you may see the various circumstances for pleasure that exist inside and around you, and happiness will flow effortlessly. Mindfulness practice should be joyful rather than laborious. Do you have to work hard to take a breath? You don't have to put up any effort. To breathe in, simply inhale. Assume you're among a group of folks watching a magnificent sunset. Do you have to make an effort to enjoy yourself?

No, you do not need to exert any effort. You simply like it. The same is true for your breath. Allow your breath to happen. Make yourself aware of it and appreciate it. Effortlessness. Enjoyment. The same is true for attentive walking. Each stride you take is pleasurable. Every step brings you closer to the wonders of life, both within and around you. Every stride is a step toward peace. Every step is a delight. That is a possibility. When you practice mindfulness, you stop talking—not only talking outside but also talking inside. The internal dialogue is the mental monologue that goes on and on and on. True quiet is the cessation of speaking—both with the lips and with the thoughts. This is not the type of quiet that enslaves us. It's a really exquisite, very strong form of quiet.

The stillness is what heals and nurtures us. Joy and pleasure are born through mindfulness. Concentration is another source of happiness. The energy of awareness carries the energy of focus within it. We say you are concentrating on the flower when you are aware of something, such as a flower, and can retain that awareness. When your awareness grows powerful, so does your concentration, and when you are totally focused, you have the opportunity to make a breakthrough, to reach insight. When you meditate on a cloud, you can get insight into its nature.

You may also concentrate on a pebble and, with appropriate attention and concentration, glimpse into the nature of the pebble. You may focus on someone and, with enough attention and concentration, you can reach a breakthrough and grasp their essence. You can focus your meditation on yourself, your wrath, your fear, your pleasure, or your tranquility.

You may meditate on anything, and with great energy of focus, you can achieve a breakthrough and acquire understanding. It acts like a magnifying glass, focusing on the sun's rays. A piece of paper will burn if you place a point of focused light on it.

Similarly, when your mindfulness and concentration are strong, your insight will free you from fear, wrath, and despair, bringing you real pleasure, peace, and contentment. The more aware and concentrated you are when contemplating the enormous, complete dawn, the more the beauty of the morning is exposed to you. Assume you are served a cup of fragrant, delicious tea. You won't be able to appreciate the tea if your mind is diverted. You must be aware of the tea and concentrate on it in order for it to show its scent and magic to you. That is why mindfulness and focus are such happy things. That is why a skilled practitioner can instill a sense of excitement and happiness at any time of day. Mindful Breathing is the first mindfulness exercise.

The first exercise is easy, but the power, or effect, might be enormous. Simply identify the in-breath as in-breath and the out-breath as out-breath during the workout. When you take a breath in, you know it's your in-breath. When you exhale, you are aware that this is your out-breath. Simply understand that this is an in-breath and this is an out-breath. Very simple and straightforward. You must return your awareness back to yourself in order to notice you're in-breath as such. Your mind is what is noticing you're in-breath, and the object of your mind—the object of your mindfulness—is the in-breath. Mindfulness is always aware of something. It's called awareness of drinking when you drink your tea attentively. Walking thoughtfully is referred to as mindfulness of walking. And mindfulness of breathing occurs when you breathe thoughtfully. So your breath is the target of your awareness, and you just focus your attention on it. Inhaling, this is my in-breath. Breathing out, this is my exhalation. When you do this, the mental dialogue will come to a halt. You no longer think. You don't have to make an effort to stop thinking; simply focus your attention on your in-breath and the mental chatter ceases. That is the practice's miracle. You no longer dwell on the past. You don't consider the future. You're not thinking about your tasks because you're concentrating your attention, your awareness, on your breathing.

It just gets better from here. You may relax and enjoy your in-breath. The practice may be enjoyable and pleasurable. A dead person cannot take any more in-breaths. But you're still alive. You are breathing in, and while doing so, you are aware that you are alive. The in-breath may be incredibly pleasant since it is a celebration of the fact that you are alive. When you are glad and happy, you do not feel the need to exert any effort. I am conscious; I am breathing in. As a result, breathing may be a celebration of life.

An in-breath might take three, four, or five seconds. That is the time to be alive, to take in your breath. You do not need to obstruct your respiration. Allow your in-breath to be brief if it is. Allow your out-breath to be as long as it has to be. Don't attempt to push it. The technique consists of just recognizing the in-breath and out-breath. That is sufficient. It will have a significant impact.

Concentration

Concentration is a wonder that you are still alive. Being alive is the greatest of all marvels, and as you breathe in, you touch that miracle. The second exercise is to track your in-breath from beginning to end while breathing in. If your in-breath is three or four seconds long, your mindfulness will be three or four seconds long as well. I take a deep breath in and follow it all the way through. When I exhale, I follow my out-breath all the way through. My thoughts are constantly with me from the beginning to the conclusion of my out-breath. As a result, awareness becomes continuous, and the quality of your attention improves. It makes no difference if they are short or long. What matters is that you follow your breath from start to finish. Your awareness is maintained. There is no pause.
Assume you're breathing in and suddenly realize, "Oh, I forgot to turn out the light in my room." There is a pause. Stick to your in-breath the entire time. Then you work on your awareness and attention. You become your in-breath. You are your out-breath. If you continue in this manner, your breathing will naturally grow deeper and slower, more harmonic and calm. It happens without any effort.

Body Awareness

The second exercise is to track your in-breath and out-breath all the way through. The final exercise is to become aware of your body when you breathe. "As I breathe in, I am conscious of my entire body." This takes it a step further.

In the first exercise, you become aware of your in-breath and out-breath. Because you have now developed the energy of attention through attentive breathing, you may utilize that energy to recognize your body.

"As I breathe in, I am conscious of my body. I'm conscious of my body when I exhale." I know my body is present. This completely reconnects the mind to the body. Mind and body merge to form one reality. When your mind is in sync with your body, you are in the present moment. You are completely awake. You may connect with the miracles of life that exist inside and around you. This practice is easy, yet the effect of body-mind unity is profound. We are rarely in that circumstance in our daily life. Our bodies are present, but our minds are elsewhere. Our minds may be caught up in the past or the future, in regrets, grief, fear, or uncertainty, and therefore our minds are not present. Someone may be there in the house, but he is not present in his head. His thoughts are on the future, on his ideas, and he is not there for his children or his marriage. Perhaps you might ask him, "Anybody home?" and assists him in returning his thoughts to his body. As a result, the third exercise is to become more conscious of your body. "I'm conscious of my body when I breathe in."
The quality of your in-breath and out-breath will improve as you practice mindful breathing. There is more peace and harmony in your breathing, and if you continue to practice in this manner, serenity and harmony will permeate the body and benefit it.

Tension Release

The following exercise can help you relax your body. When you are completely aware of your body, you will experience some tightness and discomfort, as well as some stress. The stress and agony have been building up for a long time, and our bodies are suffering as a result, but our minds are not there to assist us to release it. As a result, learning how to release tension in the body is critical. It is always feasible to remove stress when sitting, reclining, or standing. Total relaxation and deep relaxation can be practiced in a sitting or lying position. You may experience tightness in your body when driving. You are impatient to arrive and dislike the time you spend driving. When you arrive at a red light, you want it to turn green so you may proceed. However, the red light might be a signal. It may serve as a reminder of the stress of wanting to arrive as soon as possible. If you recognize it, you can utilize the red light. You can sit back and relax for 10 seconds while the light is red to practice mindful breathing and relieve tension in your body.

So next time you're stopped at a red light, you might like to sit back and do the fourth exercise: "Breathing in, I'm conscious of my body. "By exhaling, I remove the stress in my body."
Peace is achievable at that moment, and it may be practiced many times during the day—at work, while driving while cooking while doing the dishes, and while watering the vegetable garden. It is always possible to practice releasing your own stress.

Walking Meditation

When practicing mindful breathing, you just let your breath occur. You become aware of it and appreciate it. Effortlessness. The same is true for attentive walking.
Every step is pleasurable. Every step brings you closer to the beauties of life. Every step is a delight. That is a possibility. Walking meditation does not need any effort since it is pleasurable. You are present, body and mind. You are totally awake and present in the here and now. With each stride, you come into contact with the miracles of life that exist inside and around you. Every stride you take like that provides healing. Because each step is a miracle, each step gives calm and joy.
The true miracle is not being able to fly or walk on fire. The true miracle is to be able to walk on Earth, and you can do so at any time. Simply return your thoughts back to your body, awaken, and execute the miracle of walking on Earth.

Stress-reducing activities

This collection of fun activities for anxious adults contains some enjoyable stress relief activities for groups as well as some wonderful stress reduction tactics for individuals. So, here's how to deal with stress in your life:

Have Fun Coloring

Coloring is no longer only for youngsters. It is, in fact, one of the most popular enjoyable stress reduction exercises for adults for relieving tension and anxiety. Coloring will help you relax by allowing you to stay in the now and concentrate on what you're doing. So, the next time you're anxious, pick out a decent coloring book and relax with a long coloring session.

Similarly, sketching is another way to de-stressing and takes a break from troubling thoughts, and this doodle deck will undoubtedly assist you!

Participate in Board Games

It's no surprise that board games are fun to play with others. You'll be relieved to know, though, that playing board games may also help reduce stress by enhancing your mood. So, schedule regular game evenings with friends and family and play your favorite board games.

Gardening Can Help You Deal With Stress

Being in nature, surrounded by greenery, is said to be one of the scientifically established methods of reducing stress. Gardening is not everyone's go-to stress-relief hobby. However, if you have a green thumb, gardening is a pleasurable pastime that may greatly enhance your mental health. Caring for houseplants may be just as soothing.

Take a Soothing Bath

Bathing in warm water is one of the most common methods for relieving tension and discomfort. Bathing has significantly more physical and mental health advantages than showering. You may also take it a step further by enjoying a relaxing bubble bath.

Listen to Some Relaxing Music

Just as uplifting music might help you get in a good mood. Slow music, on the other hand, enables you to rest and de-stress. You may listen to music while lying on the sofa doing nothing, or you can listen to music in the background as you work.

Adult Stress-Relieving Toys

Stress relief toys are excellent for fidgeting. And having a desk toy is one of the most basic methods to reduce stress at work. In fact, most fidget toys are small enough to bring with you wherever you go.

Take a Deep Breath

A healthy mind and body are required for productive employment. Work-related burnout, on the other hand, might have a negative impact on your health. That's when you should think about taking a day (or two) off. Everyone needs a break from time to time, whether it's a short one or a longer one, to rest and rejuvenate.

Dance as though no one is looking

If physical activity isn't your thing, dancing can be. Dancing not only keeps you physically active, but it also improves your mood. So, when you're too tired to do anything else, put on your favorite music and dance like no one is looking!!

Stress Relieving Aromatherapy

Aromatherapy is the technique of employing fragrant materials to improve one's health in general. Essential oils are becoming increasingly popular for use in aromatherapy. They may be used to address a variety of issues in a variety of ways (including stress and anxiety). Furthermore, they are extremely simple and convenient to use.
You may also relax by lighting a relaxing scented candle. It will assist you in bringing warmth into your house after a long day.

Laugh more frequently

"Laughter is the best medicine," as they say, and a good belly laugh actually cures and relaxes your body. On social media, you may occasionally view humorous films or movies or go through some hilarious memes. Spending time with your pets or having fun with your loved ones may also help to relieve stress.

Mindfulness Meditation for Stress

One of the most basic stress-relieving exercises for adults is meditation. At first, it may appear frightening. Anyone, with practice, can do it.
If you're just getting started, guided meditations will be quite beneficial. Begin with 10 minutes and gradually increase your time.

Learn to Knit

Knitting may be a passion for some, but did you know it has various health benefits?! So, if you enjoy crafts and are seeking for a creative pastime to release stress, knitting is the way to go!! It's comparable to mindfulness methods in that it helps with anxiety, stress, and sadness.

Get Moving to Deal with Stress

Do you think you're too busy to fit physical activity into your everyday routine? Consider again!!
A little exercise goes a long way when it comes to consistently managing stress!! If you like sports, you may also try out numerous sporting activities.

Begin with Stress Cleaning for Self-Solution

One of my favorite ways to relieve tension! Yes, stress-cleaning works and is quite soothing. Consider cleaning as a kind of self-care if you don't particularly love it. Furthermore, it does not imply that you must clean your entire house at once. Begin with little chores and work your way up. Even the most basic tasks will help.

Organize Your Sleep Schedule

When you're overly worried and nothing else appears to be working, all you need is a good night's sleep. Stress and worry, on the other

hand, can induce sleep issues, making it difficult to obtain a decent night's sleep. To address the fundamental problem, you must practice proper sleep hygiene and modify your nighttime routine.
Furthermore, if you believe you are not receiving enough sleep on a regular basis. Try sleeping for an extra hour or increasing your sleep time. It will have a big influence on your general way of living.

WHAT IS THE DEFINITION OF EMOTIONAL SELF-CARE?

Emotional self-care is a strategy for recognizing and nurturing one's feelings, perceptions, and thoughts in order to improve emotional well-being. It is one of five distinct types of self-care practices that will help you satisfy your emotional needs.

Emotional self-care activities, on the other hand, do not ensure that you will always be happy; rather, they assist you in accepting all of your feelings, both positive and bad.

The Importance of Emotional Self-Care

Your emotions, whether happy or unpleasant, are what define you as a person.

Fear allows you to live in the worst-case situation, whereas discomfort alerts you to the presence of a problem, and assertiveness helps you to take decisive action and make judgments. Emotions naturally assist us in engaging with people.

Overall, emotions contribute to identifying problems that require your attention. As a result, emotional self-care is essential for your emotional health.

The Benefits of Emotional Self-Care

Emotional self-care helps with stress management as well as mental health issues like depression and anxiety. It also helps with mental

recovery after terrible experiences including severe childhood traumas and physical abuse.
As a result, dealing with the stress and concern that have become ordinary in our everyday lives necessitates emotional self-care.

Here's a self-help guide on emotional self-care that offers some suggestions for coping with your mental health when things become rough.

Establish healthy limits

Healthy boundaries are self-imposed restraints. It will determine the acceptable behavior of others around you, as well as how you will react when those limits are violated. They might be both physical and emotional in nature. Setting solid boundaries is critical for safeguarding your time, values, and safety, as well as your emotional well-being.

Master the Art of Saying NO

Saying NO is part of establishing healthy boundaries. It will empower you while also actively supporting you in keeping your connections.
As a result, practice saying NO politely and without apologizing.

Recognition

As you are undoubtedly aware, we have very little control over many aspects of our lives, including our emotions. And we all go through times when negativity overwhelms us and puts us powerless. Accepting such events as they are is therefore essential for dealing with them. It will save you a significant amount of time and work.

Allow yourself the freedom to let go

You're not alone if you can't decide whether to cling on or let go. We all retain things for a longer period of time than we should. There are instances, though, when letting go is the greatest thing you can do for yourself. Allow yourself to let go of things that no longer serve you. Otherwise, it will restrict your growth.

Forgiveness of oneself

Forgiving yourself for prior mistakes would assist you in getting rid of your guilt and regrets. It will also allow you to focus more on the present circumstance. Furthermore, guilt has significant health consequences that are not always obvious. As a result, self-forgiveness is essential for moving forward in life in a healthy way.

Before retiring to bed, express gratitude

Practicing gratitude trains you to see the positive in everything, which is a strong habit to cultivate. And posting about gratitude is the simplest way to end the day on a positive note.

Leave

People frequently fail to see that this alternative is constantly available. You don't have to always put on a pleasant front. It is perfectly OK to leave any situation that makes you feel uncomfortable, lonely, or sad, whether it be a party or any other situation in which you do not feel like you belong.

Accept your feelings

You may feel guilty at times, but this is not a sensible problem to tackle. Furthermore, your unhappiness may be impeding your progress in life.
Rather than trying to ignore or control your emotions, aim to accept them. It will allow you to handle them appropriately.

Make an effort to prevent negative self-talk

Self-criticism and pathological perfectionism promote negative self-talk. It is tough to remain optimistic under such circumstances. Instead of being judgmental of yourself, accept your flaws. You may also develop healthy lifestyle habits such as positive self-talk and body language. It will encourage you to focus on the positive aspects of your life rather than the negative.

Disconnect everything

While technology facilitates socialization, it may also make you feel self-conscious. Instead of entirely avoiding it, think about withdrawing from time to time.

Bullet Journal

Making a list of what makes you happy is a fun way to exercise self-care while keeping organized.

A bullet notebook can help you with habit tracking, mood tracking, goal planning, and organizing your life in a more visually pleasing manner, in addition to writing activities.

Vision board for visualization

Visualization, in combination with a vision board, is a very effective self-care method. A vision board is a flat panel containing an inspiring collection of slogans, photos, and other stuff. It's a fantastic way to stay motivated, whether you're caring for yourself or striving to reach your goals.

Idea generation

The practice of clearing your mind is known as brain dumping. It enables you to send stray thoughts from your head to a journal or notes app on your phone for subsequent review.

This can help you free some mental space and reduce your anxiety.

Play some music

Music has the power to be both healing and enjoyable. Create a playlist to help you get in the mood. It will provide meaning to the time spent listening to music.

Schedule time for isolation

It is a luxury to have some peace and quiet in the midst of an unexpected and frantic living. So, wherever possible, make time for yourself in the middle of your daily activities.

Make touch with someone you care about

Speak with someone you care about, whether it's a friend, family member, or someone else. It might be a phone call, a text message, or any other manner that you like. It may help you feel better in any situation.

Simply put on a happy face

A simple grin may mislead your brain into thinking you're pleased, which can help relieve anxiety. So have a smile on your face at all times! If you can't, try putting on a fake smile until you can.

Using positive affirmations

A practice of repeating your affirmations may help you deal with practically any negative scenario. Just make sure your remarks are not illogical, but rather something in which you believe. You may maintain motivating and positive design products about your house, office, or workstation to keep you inspired at all times. Reading is a great way to stay motivated and informed. It doesn't matter if the book is fictional or nonfiction. In addition to books, you may read self-help articles, journals, and even blogs.

Express Your Emotions

Share your thoughts and concerns with those you can rely on. It can help you cope with problems more effectively. The more you open up about your problems to others, the more they will open up to you.

Fidgeting gadgets

Sensory fidget toys may either help or hamper your concentration. They are perfect for people with work-related stress, anxiety, ADHD, or other fidgeting issues. Toys such as fidget spinners, stress balls, and infinity cubes are trendy these days. There are also several imaginative and engaging sensory fidget toys on the market that are appropriate for both youngsters and adults.

Fika

Fika is the Swedish custom of taking a daily coffee break. It is, however, much more than just grabbing a cup of coffee. It is about taking a break from the hectic pace of daily life and slowing down to enjoy a simple pleasure (drinking coffee or tea).

Reward yourself

When everything else fails, PAMPER YOURSELF!!! This is one of the most effective yet unappreciated forms of self-care. There are times in life when nothing feels right. That is when you need to be pampered. Pampering oneself is a guaranteed way to relieve stress and anxiety.

There are several ways to reward oneself, and it may be as simple as watching your favorite show on Netflix.

I hope these tips have motivated you to easily engage in emotional self-care practices when life becomes rough.

CHAPTER 4

Sleep is a necessary function that helps your body and mind to replenish, allowing you to wake up refreshed and aware. A good night's sleep also helps the body stay healthy and avoid ailments. The brain cannot operate correctly if it does not get adequate sleep. This can affect your ability to focus, think effectively, and recall memories.

Most individuals require between seven and nine hours of sleep every night. Children and teens require much more sleep, especially if they are under the age of five. Work schedules, daily worries, a noisy bedroom environment, and medical issues can all interfere with getting adequate sleep. A balanced diet and excellent living choices can help guarantee that you get enough sleep each night, but for some people, persistent sleep deprivation is the first indicator of a sleep problem.

THE SCIENCE OF SLEEP

An internal "body clock" governs your sleep cycle, determining when you are weary and ready for bed, as well as when you are refreshed and awake. The circadian rhythm is a 24-hour cycle that this clock follows. You will grow progressively fatigued during the day after waking up from sleep. These emotions will peak in the evening before bedtime.

This sleep drive, also known as sleep-wake homeostasis, may be connected to adenosine, a brain-produced chemical molecule. Adenosine levels rise during the day as you feel fatigued, and the body breaks it down during sleep.

The circadian rhythm is also influenced by light. The hypothalamus is a particular area of nerve cells in the brain, and it contains a cluster of cells called the suprachiasmatic nucleus, which processes signals when the eyes are exposed to natural or artificial light. These signals assist the brain in determining whether or not it is day or night.

As natural light fades in the evening, the body produces melatonin, a drowsiness-inducing hormone. When the sun rises in the morning, the body produces cortisol, a hormone that promotes energy and alertness.

Sleeping Stages

Once we fall asleep, our bodies go through a four-stage sleep cycle. Non-rapid eye movement (NREM) sleep is the first three phases, while rapid eye movement (REM) sleep is the fourth stage.

• Stage 1 NREM: This initial stage, which comprises of light sleep, symbolizes the transition between awake and sleep. Muscles relax, and your heart rate, breathing, and eye movements, as well as your brain waves, which are more active while you are awake, begin to calm down. Stage 1 usually lasts a few minutes.

• Stage 2 NREM: This second NREM sleep stage is characterized by deeper slumber as your heart rate and breathing rate continue to drop down and your muscles relax. Your eye movements will stop and your body temperature will drop. Aside from a few transient bursts of higher frequency electrical activity, brain waves remain sluggish. Stage 2 is usually the longest of the four sleep stages.

• Stage 3 NREM: This stage is critical in helping you feel refreshed and awake the next day. Heart rate, respiration, and brain wave activity all reach their lowest levels, and the muscles are as relaxed as they will be. This stage will be lengthier at first and then shorten during the night.

• REM: The first REM period occurs around 90 minutes after you fall asleep. As the name implies, your eyes will travel back and forth fast beneath your eyelids. The pace of breathing, heart rate, and blood pressure will begin to rise. Dreaming usually occurs during REM sleep, and your arms and legs will go paralyzed - this is thought to protect you from physically acting out your dreams. As the night passes, the duration of each REM sleep cycle rises. REM sleep has also been related to memory consolidation, the process of transforming freshly learned experiences into long-term memories, according to several research. As you become older, the duration of the REM stage shortens, forcing you to spend more time in the NREM phases.

These four stages will cycle through your night till you wake up. Each cycle will take around 90-120 minutes for most folks. NREM sleep accounts for around 75% to 80% of each cycle. You may sometimes wake up momentarily throughout the night but have no recollection of what happened the next day. These are referred to as "W" phases.

The Importance of Adequate Sleep

Most individuals require at least seven hours of sleep every night for optimum cognitive and behavioral functions. An inadequate quantity of sleep might have catastrophic consequences. According to several research, sleep deprivation makes people more prone to attention lapses, impaired cognition, delayed reactions, and mood swings.

It's also been hypothesized that persistent sleep deprivation might cause people to acquire a type of tolerance. Even though their minds and bodies are suffering as a result of a lack of sleep, people may be unaware of their own limitations because less sleep feels normal to them. Furthermore, a lack of sleep has been related to an increased risk of various illnesses and medical disorders. Obesity, type 2 diabetes, high blood pressure, heart disease, stroke, poor mental health, and premature mortality are among them.

Adults who do not get enough sleep each night might change their lifestyle and sleep patterns to get the necessary seven to nine hours of sleep. These are some examples:

• Set a reasonable bedtime and adhere to it every night, including on weekends.

• Keep your bedroom at a reasonable temperature and with low lighting levels.

• Maintain a pleasant sleeping environment by using the finest mattress, pillows, and sheets for your sleep preferences and body type.

• Consider imposing a "screen ban" in your bedroom on televisions, laptops and tablets, mobile phones, and other electronic gadgets.

• Avoid caffeine, alcohol, and heavy meals in the hours before night.

• Avoid using cigarettes at any time of day or night.

• Exercising during the day might help you relax and prepare for sleep in the evening.

• Sleep should be restful, yet 35% of people struggle to acquire the required seven or more hours of sleep every night. Given the potential implications of not getting enough sleep, such as decreased performance and an increased risk of cardiovascular disease, cancer, diabetes, high blood pressure, and vehicle accidents, it's no wonder that many individuals resort to sleep aids to help them sleep.

Natural sleep aids are becoming increasingly popular as an alternative to prescription and over-the-counter medications. Educating yourself about the many types of natural sleep aids, their possible advantages and drawbacks, and how they are regulated will assist you in making educated decisions about using and purchasing these items.

What Are Circadian Rhythms?

Circadian rhythms are 24-hour cycles that operate in the background to carry out key tasks and processes. The sleep-wake cycle is a well-known and significant circadian rhythm.

Circadian rhythms are followed by many systems of the body and are synced with a master clock in the brain. Because this master clock is strongly regulated by environmental stimuli, particularly light, circadian rhythms are linked to the day-night cycle.
A circadian cycle, when correctly aligned, can promote regular and restorative sleep. When this circadian cycle is disrupted, it can cause serious sleeping issues, including insomnia. Circadian rhythms, according to research, play an important role in many areas of physical and mental health.

What Is Circadian Rhythm and How Does It Work?

Circadian rhythms function by ensuring that the body's operations are optimal at various moments over a 24-hour period. Circadian is derived from the Latin phrase "circa diem," which means "about a day."

Circadian rhythms may be found in all species. For example, they assist flowers in opening and closing at the appropriate times and prevent nocturnal creatures from leaving their refuge during the day, when they would be vulnerable to more predators.

Circadian rhythms in humans regulate mental and bodily processes throughout the body. The digestive system generates proteins to correspond with average meal time, while the endocrine system controls hormones to correspond with regular energy expenditure.

The circadian rhythms of the body are linked to a master clock, also known as the circadian pacemaker, which is housed in the brain. It is specifically present in the suprachiasmatic nucleus (SCN), which is located in the hypothalamus region of the brain. Clock genes in the SCN deliver signals to control activity throughout the body at different times of the day.

The SCN is extremely light sensitive, and light acts as an important external cue that modulates the signals transmitted by the SCN to coordinate internal clocks in the body. As a result, circadian rhythms are inextricably linked to day and night. While other signals such as exercise, social interaction, and temperature can impact the master clock, light has the greatest influence on circadian rhythms.

What Is the Difference Between a Circadian Rhythm and a Biological Clock?

Biological clocks aid in the timing of biological activities such as circadian cycles. A circadian rhythm is a biological clock effect, however not all biological clocks are circadian. Plants, for example, respond to changing seasons by employing a biological clock with timing that differs from a 24-hour cycle.

What Effect Does Circadian Rhythm Have on Sleep?

When individuals discuss circadian rhythm, they usually refer to sleep. One of the most obvious and fundamental examples of the relevance of circadian rhythms is the sleep-wake cycle.

During the day, light exposure stimulates the master clock to transmit signals that create awareness and aid in keeping us awake and active. As night falls, the master clock starts producing

melatonin, a hormone that promotes sleep, and then continues to
send signals that help us sleep through the night.

As a result, our circadian rhythm matches our sleep and wakefulness
with day and night, resulting in a steady cycle of restorative rest that
allows for more daytime activity.

Aside from sleep, what else does Circadian Rhythm affect?

While the sleep-wake cycle is one of the most well-known circadian
rhythms, these 24-hour internal clocks play an important part in
almost all of the body's functions.

Although research on circadian rhythms is ongoing, evidence has
linked them to metabolism and weight through the regulation of
blood sugar and cholesterol. Circadian rhythms also have an impact
on mental health, including the risk of psychiatric illnesses such as
depression and bipolar disorder, as well as the risk of
neurodegenerative diseases such as dementia.
There is evidence that circadian rhythms have a significant impact
on the immune system as well as DNA repair mechanisms involved
in cancer prevention. Early research suggests that circadian cycles
might impact the efficacy of anti-cancer treatments, and that future
therapies may be able to use biological clocks to destroy cancer
cells.

What Happens When the Circadian Rhythm Is Out of Sync?

When the circadian rhythm is disrupted, the body's processes do not
work efficiently.

A disrupted sleep-wake circadian cycle can lead to major sleeping
issues. A person may struggle to fall asleep, wake up during the
night, or be unable to sleep as long as they desire into the morning if
their body's internal clock is not properly signaled. Their overall
amount of sleep may be decreased, and a disturbed circadian rhythm
may result in shallower, fragmented, and lower-quality sleep.

Furthermore, studies have implicated circadian rhythm abnormalities as potential factors to snoring, a sleep condition characterized by frequent gaps in breathing. OSA depletes the body's oxygen levels and disrupts sleep throughout the night.

A misaligned circadian rhythm can have a detrimental impact on sleep in a variety of ways, including an increased risk of insomnia and excessive daytime drowsiness. Given the importance of sleep for productivity and general health, disruptions in a person's circadian rhythm can have serious implications.

What Factors Can Affect Circadian Rhythm?

Circadian rhythm disruptions can occur in the short or long term. Based on their features and causes, experts have classified circadian rhythm sleep-wake disorders (CRSWD) into many categories.

• **Jet Lag Disorder**: This happens when a person crosses many time zones in a short period of time and is named from the fact that it is frequently encountered by those who fly across continents. Sleeping issues and exhaustion from jet lag are probable until a person's circadian rhythm adjusts to the day-night cycle of their new location.

• **Shift Work Disorder**: Work duties can significantly alter a person's circadian rhythm. Shift employment, which demands working through the night and sleeping throughout the day, directly contradicts a person's sleep cycle with the local daylight hours.

• **Advanced Sleep Phase Disorder**: People with this disorder get fatigued early in the evening and wake up quite early in the morning. People with advanced sleep phase disorders typically cannot stay awake later at night or sleep later in the morning. This condition is quite uncommon, affecting around 1% of persons in their middle and later years, and it is more common in older adults. Advanced sleep phase disorder may have a hereditary genetic basis in some circumstances.

• **Delayed Sleep Phase Disorder**: "night owls" who stay up late at night and sleep in late in the morning are prone to this sort of circadian rhythm disturbance. It is uncommon in the general population, affecting just one or two persons out of every 1,000, but it affects up to 16% of teenagers. The precise reason is unknown, however it might be linked to heredity, underlying medical issues, and a person's behavior.

• **Non-24 Hour Sleep Wake Disorder**: This disorder typically affects blind persons who are unable to receive light-based cues for their circadian rhythm. Their body still operates on a 24-hour cycle, but their sleeping hours are continuously shifting backward by minutes or hours.

• **Irregular Sleep-Wake Rhythm Disorder**: People with this unusual disorder have no constant sleep pattern and may take multiple naps or have brief intervals of sleep during a 24-hour day. It is usually linked to brain diseases, such as dementia or traumatic brain injury, that impair the correct operation of the master clock in the hypothalamus.

There are several reasons of circadian rhythm problems, as seen by this list. Some circadian disturbances are caused by individual action, such as travel or job, which causes sleep cycles to be out of sync with regular daylight exposure. Other diseases are caused by an underlying problem that prevents the body's master clock from receiving or processing external stimuli. In certain cases, hereditary reasons may be implicated, or the cause may be unknown.

Maintaining a Healthy Circadian Rhythm

While we don't have complete control over our circadian rhythm, there are certain healthy sleep strategies we may try to better entrain our 24-hour sleep cycles.

• Seek out natural light: Exposure to natural light, particularly early in the day, helps reinforce the strongest circadian signal.

• Stick to a constant sleep schedule: Changing your bedtime or morning wake-up time might make it difficult for your body to acclimatize to a steady circadian rhythm.

• Engage in regular physical activity: Physical activity throughout the day might boost your internal clock and make it simpler to fall asleep at night.

• Stay away from caffeine: Caffeine and other stimulants can keep you awake and disrupt the normal balance of sleep and alertness. Everyone is different, but if you're having difficulty sleeping, avoid coffee after midday.
• Limit light exposure before bed: Artificial light exposure at night might disrupt the circadian cycle. Experts recommend lowering the lights and putting electronic gadgets away before night, as well as keeping electronics out of the bedroom and away from your mattress.

• Take brief, early-afternoon naps: Late and extended naps might push back your bedtime and throw your sleep routine off.

These actions to enhance sleep hygiene can help promote a healthy circadian rhythm, although extra measures may be required depending on the scenario. If you experience persistent or severe sleeping issues, daytime tiredness, and/or a troublesome sleep routine, it's critical to consult with a doctor who can best evaluate the reason and provide the best therapy.

Dreams are one of the most enthralling and perplexing components of sleep. Since Sigmund Freud helped call attention to the potential relevance of dreams in the late nineteenth century, significant study has been conducted to uncover both the neuroscience and psychology of dreams.
Despite advances in scientific understanding, much about sleep and dreams remains unclear. Even the most fundamental issue — why do we dream at all? — is still hotly debated.

While everyone dreams, the substance of those dreams and their impact on sleep might differ greatly amongst people. Even though there is no easy explanation for the meaning and purpose of dreams, understanding the fundamentals of dreams, the possible impact of nightmares, and measures you may take to sleep better with lovely dreams is beneficial.

What Exactly Are Dreams?

Dreams are sights, thoughts, or sensations experienced while sleeping. The most common is visual imagery, although dreams can encompass all of the senses. Some people experience colour dreams, while others have black and white dreams, and others who are blind have more dream components relating to sound, taste, and smell. Various studies have found various sorts of dream content, however some common dream qualities include:

• It is involuntary and features a first-person perspective.

• The material might be nonsensical, if not incoherent.

• Other individuals engage with the dreamer and with one another in the content.

• It elicits intense emotions.

• Aspects of daily life are interwoven into the text.

Although these characteristics are not ubiquitous, they may be seen in most regular dreams to some level.

WHAT MAKES US DREAM?

Sleep researchers continue to debate why we dream. Among the several theories concerning the function of dreaming are:
• Memory consolidation: Dreaming has been linked to memory consolidation, suggesting that it may serve an essential cognitive role of improving memory and informative recall.

• Emotion processing: The ability to engage with and rehearse emotions in various imagined scenarios may be part of the brain's mechanism for controlling emotions.

• Mental housekeeping: Dreaming may be the brain's way of "straightening out," removing incomplete, incorrect, or superfluous information.

• Dream material may be a type of warped instant replay in which recent events are examined and assessed.

• Incidental brain activity: According to this viewpoint, dreaming is only a byproduct of sleep with no inherent function or significance.

Neuroscientists and psychologists continue to undertake tests to determine what happens in the brain during sleep, but even with continued study, it may be hard to verify any explanation for why we dream.

WHEN DO WE SLEEP?

Most people dream for about two hours every night on average. Dreams can occur at any stage of sleep, but they are most frequent and powerful during the rapid eye movement (REM) period.

Brain activity increases significantly during the REM sleep stage compared to the non-REM phases, which helps to explain the different forms of dreaming that occur throughout various stages. Even while they may contain elements of everyday life, dreams during REM sleep are often more vivid, fanciful, and/or weird. Non-REM dreams, on the other hand, tend to have more cohesive content, such as ideas or memories tied to a certain time and location.

REM sleep is not equally dispersed throughout the night. The majority of REM sleep occurs in the second half of a typical sleep cycle, therefore dreaming is focused in the hours before waking up.

DO YOUR DREAMS HAVE ANY MEANING?

Dream interpretation and if they have any meaning at all are hotly debated topics. While some psychologists believe that dreams can give insight into a person's psychology or daily life, others believe that their content is too inconsistent or perplexing to dependably convey significance.

Almost all specialists agree that dreams can contain material that is related to waking events, albeit the content may be altered or misinterpreted. In discussing dreams, for example, individuals frequently refer to persons they recognize even though their appearance is altered in the dream.

The relevance of real-life information appearing in dreams, on the other hand, is far from clear. According to the "continuity theory" in dream study, dreams and waking life are connected and so entail overlapping.

The relevance of real-life information appearing in dreams, on the other hand, is far from clear. In dream study, the "continuity hypothesis" states that dreams and waking life are interwoven and hence feature overlapping themes and substance. The "discontinuity theory," on the other hand, regards dream and wakeful thought as fundamentally separate.

While dream analysis may be a component of personal or psychological self-reflection, there is no clear method for interpreting and comprehending the significance of dreams in waking, everyday life based on available information.

WHAT ARE THE DIFFERENT TYPES OF DREAMS?

Dreams may manifest themselves in a variety of ways. Lucid dreams happen when a person is in a dream yet is fully aware that they are dreaming. Dream material in vivid dreams is extremely realistic or clear. Bad dreams include upsetting or painful material. The same imagery appears in several dreams throughout time in recurring nightmares.

Even in ordinary dreams, there are some sorts of material that are easily identified. Things like flying, falling, being followed, or being unable to find a restroom are among the most identifiable and typical motifs in dreams.

WHAT EXACTLY ARE NIGHTMARES?

A nightmare is a horrible dream that causes a person to wake up from sleep, according to sleep medicine. This term differs from normal use, which refers to any dangerous, frightening, or annoying dream as a nightmare. While disturbing dreams are typical and usually harmless, repeated nightmares can disrupt sleep and cause poor thinking and mood throughout the day.

DO DREAMS INFLUENCE SLEEP?

Dreams seldom interfere with sleep. Dreaming is a natural element of sleep and is typically regarded as entirely normal and without any detrimental impacts on sleep.

The only exception is nightmares. Because nightmares entail awakenings, they can be distressing if they happen frequently. Disturbing dreams may drive a person to avoid sleep, resulting in inadequate sleep. When they do sleep, the previous sleep deprivation might cause a REM sleep rebound, which can exacerbate nightmares. Because of this negative loop, some people who have frequent nightmares may develop insomnia as a persistent sleep condition.

As a result, those who suffer nightmares more than once a week, sleep fragmentation, daytime tiredness, or changes in their thinking or mood should consult a doctor. A doctor can examine these symptoms to determine the possible reasons and therapies for their sleeping disorder.

HOW DO YOU RECALL YOUR DREAMS?

Remembering dreams is an important first step for persons who desire to document or analyze them. The capacity to recall dreams differs from person to person and may alter with age. While there is no certain strategy to increase dream recollection, experts offer the following strategies:

• As soon as you wake up, consider your dreams. Dreams may be lost in the blink of an eye, so make remembering them your top priority when you wake up. Close your eyes and attempt to relive your dreams in your head before sitting up or even saying good morning to your bed companion.

• Keep a diary or an app on hand to keep track of your dream material. It's critical to have a strategy for swiftly recording dream details before forgetting them, especially if you wake up in the middle of the night. Most individuals find keeping a pen and paper on their nightstand works well, but there are smart phone applications that may help you construct an organized and searchable dream journal.

• Try to wake up gently in the morning. An rapid awakening, such as from an alarm clock, may lead you to startle up and out of a dream, making it difficult to remember the contents.

• Remind yourself that remembering your dreams is important. Tell yourself that you will recall your dreams in the days leading up to night, and repeat this mantra before going to sleep. While this cannot guarantee that you will remember your dreams, it can help you remember to take the time to meditate on them before beginning your day.

HOW CAN YOU GET RID OF NIGHTMARES?

People who have frequent nightmares that disrupt their sleep should see a doctor so that they can be diagnosed with nightmare disorder or another ailment impacting their sleep quality. Treatment for nightmare disorder frequently includes talk therapy, which aims to overcome negative thinking, tension, and worry, all of which can exacerbate nightmares.

Many forms of talk therapy aim to alleviate anxieties or fears, including those that may emerge during dreams. Because just suppressing bad ideas may increase nightmares, this form of exposure or desensitization treatment helps many patients reframe their emotional reaction to unwanted images.
Improving sleep hygiene, which encompasses both sleep-related routines and the bedroom environment, is another step toward reducing nightmares. Healthy sleep hygiene can help you sleep better even if you experience disturbing nightmares by making your nightly sleep more regular. Healthy sleep suggestions include:

• Maintain a consistent sleep pattern: Maintain a consistent schedule every day, even weekends and other days when you don't have to get up at a specific hour.

• Select pre-bed material with care: Avoid scary, unpleasant, or exciting stuff in the hours before bed since it may cause negative thoughts during sleeping.

• Unwind at the end of each day: Exercising throughout the day might help you sleep better at night. Allow your mind and body to peacefully relax before bedtime, such as by gentle stretching, deep breathing, or other relaxation techniques.

• Limit alcohol and caffeine: Alcohol use might lead to more concentrated REM sleep later in the night, increasing the chance of nightmares. Caffeine is a stimulant that can disrupt your sleep cycle and keep your brain charged even when you want to sleep.

• Keep distractions out of the bedroom: Create a sleeping environment that is dark, quiet, smells great, and is at a suitable temperature. A comfortable mattress and pillow may make your bed more appealing. All of these characteristics make it easier to remain calm and avoid uncomfortable awakenings, which can lead to inconsistent sleep patterns.

WHAT EXACTLY ARE NATURAL SLEEP AIDS?

• Natural sleep aids are over-the-counter supplements designed to help you fall asleep sooner or remain asleep all night. They are often plant-based, a vitamin or mineral already present in our meals, or additional levels of something created by the body. There are no precise restrictions for the usage of the term "natural" for supplements, and many natural supplements, such as melatonin, are synthetically generated. Many clients prefer natural sleep pills because they have fewer adverse effects than prescription sleep drugs. They also appeal to consumers who prefer natural goods or are concerned about the addictive potential of pharmaceutical sleep aids.

• The US Food and Drug Administration does not regularly monitor the safety and efficacy of supplements (FDA). Shoppers should take extra precautions to ensure they are acquiring trusted items.

NATURAL SLEEP SUPPLEMENTS

There is a dizzying assortment of natural sleep aids available, many of which promise to provide the rest you require. Learning about the science behind various supplements, as well as their possible adverse effects, might help you select which natural sleep aid is ideal for you.

It is, nevertheless, vital to see your doctor before beginning any new supplement. Natural does not necessarily imply that it is safe for everyone. Many supplements are not recommended for those who have particular sensitivities or diseases, or who are taking other drugs.

Melatonin

Melatonin is a sleep-regulating hormone generated by our brain's pineal gland. It is important in the organization of our circadian rhythms, which are the 24-hour sleep-wake cycles that regulate when we get up, feel alert, weary, and sleep.

A variety of variables, mainly nighttime light exposure, but also age and other disorders, can reduce melatonin synthesis. Because low melatonin levels can disrupt sleep, many people take supplementary melatonin in tablet form. It is the fourth most popular natural supplement among adults in the United States.

Melatonin is most commonly prescribed to persons who have circadian rhythm disorders such as delayed sleep-wake phase disorder or whose circadian rhythms are disrupted by jet lag. It is also used to treat some sleep abnormalities in youngsters. Melatonin may also assist with shift work-related sleep disorders or insomnia, however data is mixed on how beneficial it is for these issues. While doctors feel that consuming regular doses of melatonin is largely safe, there are possible safety issues for youngsters.

Furthermore, allergic responses are likely, and there is little information on its usage by pregnant or nursing women. Although the side effects are not usually severe, they may include dizziness, nausea, and headaches. Some people, particularly elderly persons, experience daytime sleepiness.

Lavender

Lavender, a beloved scented garden and kitchen herb, has long been regarded to help with relaxation and sleep. Some of these traditional beliefs appear to be validated by modern study. Lavender oil, for example, has been demonstrated to improve postpartum sleep quality and boost the effectiveness of excellent sleep hygiene. Lavender oil appears to have a relaxing effect and might help with anxiety and restlessness.

The majority of research on lavender's effectiveness as a sleep aid has concentrated on lavender essential oil, while some individuals use the dried herb as a tea or in their pillow. Essential oils should only be consumed under the direction of a specialist, as even lavender oil contains toxic chemicals. Instead, disperse the oil into the air or dilute it in a neutral cream or oil for application on the skin.

Lavender may be especially enticing to persons who have trouble sleeping due to anxiousness or racing thoughts. It is also popular with folks who prefer an external sleep aid over anything they ingest. Short-term usage of dried lavender or lavender essential oil is regarded to be safe; nevertheless, potential negative effects of external lavender oil use include skin irritation and allergic response.

Valerian

Since the 2nd century, the pungent valerian herb — whose fragrance has been compared to gym socks — has been used to treat sleep disorders. Although more study is needed, valerian appears to help people fall asleep faster, sleep better, and wake up less frequently. In other trials, patients using valerian were 80% more likely than those receiving a placebo to report sleep benefits. Because no one active molecule has been identified, scientists suggest that the impact of valerian may be attributable to a combination of chemicals, or the amino acids GABA or glycine.

The valerian plant's roots and stems are used to make teas, tinctures, capsules, extracts, and pills. While each method has its supporters, the tea can have a disagreeable odor, and researchers typically employ liquid extracts or capsules in their studies. Valerian is typically prescribed for those who suffer from insomnia or other sleep-related issues. Most individuals claim that it becomes more effective after many weeks of use. More study is needed, however, to assess how beneficial valerian is in treating insomnia.

Valerian is usually thought to be safe for adults. The most common and minor side effects include headache, dizziness, itching, and stomach trouble.

Chamomile

Since ancient Egypt, German chamomile has been used to treat sleep disorders. Despite its extensive history, little study on its advantages has been conducted. What we do know from smaller trials and meta-analyses is that German chamomile may reduce anxiety and enhance sleep quality, though experts aren't sure why. On the other side, it does not appear to help persons who suffer from insomnia.

German chamomile is most often available in capsules, tincture, and tea form. Although there is another kind known as Roman chamomile, the majority of study has concentrated on the German variety.

Chamomile is typically viewed as harmless when either orally or as a tea. It may interact with several medicines, particularly blood thinners, and there is limited evidence on its safety for pregnant or nursing women. The most common side effects are moderate nausea and dizziness, although allergic responses are possible, especially in persons who are sensitive to related plants like ragweed and daisies.

Passionflower

The passionflower vine is indigenous to the Americas and has long been used as a sedative by many traditional tribes. There has been relatively little study into its advantages, yet what there is is positive, if restricted. Passionflower's soothing effects were equivalent to a regularly prescribed sedative in one research on generalized anxiety disorder. Passionflower may also increase sleep quality and make falling and staying asleep simpler.

People commonly consume passionflower extracts and tea. Both have been employed in research settings, so which one to select is a question of personal taste. While research on this supplement suggests that it may help with anxiety and sleeplessness, there is no definitive evidence of its effectiveness.

As with the advantages of passionflower, there has been minimal study on its safety. Daily dosages of up to 800 mg, however, have been used successfully in trials lasting up to two months. The most common side effects include sleepiness, disorientation, and uncoordinated movements. Passionflower should not be used by pregnant women since it might cause uterine contractions. There has been little study on its safety when nursing.

Hops In addition to being the primary flavor in beer, some individuals utilize the blooms of the hops plant as a natural sleep aid. Hops, like other natural supplements, has not been thoroughly tested to determine whether or not it can help individuals sleep better. However, preliminary research suggests that hops supplements might help regulate circadian rhythms and alleviate the symptoms of shift work disorder. Hops blossoms contain the acids humulone and lupulone, and their interaction with the body's GABA receptors may contribute to hops' effects.

Hops

Hops is frequently coupled with other natural sleep aids like valerian. It can be consumed as a non-alcoholic beer or dried as a tea or dry extract. Various research have employed all three strategies, and there is no indication that one strategy is superior to the others. Hops are likely safe to take in the form of non-alcoholic beer or tea, but supplementary usage is only deemed maybe safe due to a lack of studies. Hops also has more possible negative effects than some other natural sleep aids. Hops is not suggested for those who are pregnant or nursing, or who have hormone-sensitive malignancies or other illnesses, because it contains modest estrogen-like effects.

Hops can also exacerbate depression. However, most people have modest side effects such as dizziness or tiredness.

81

CANNABIDIOL

CBD is a substance found in the cannabis plant known as a cannabinoids. CBD differs significantly from the psychoactive delta-9-tetrahydrocannabinol (THC) cannabinoids found in cannabis. The majority of CBD is obtained from hemp, which contains little THC to be psychoactive.

CBD research has been restricted in the past owing to cannabis prohibitions, but there are evidence that it may help certain individuals sleep better. To begin, it appears to alleviate the nervous symptoms of a wide range of mental health issues. It also appears that the body's natural cannabinoids system influences how we sleep, increasing the likelihood that CBD would be beneficial. There is some evidence that CBD can help with some sleep problems and reduce excessive daytime drowsiness, although research is still preliminary.

Although CBD has been allowed in the United States since 2018, it is not permitted to be sold as a dietary supplement. However, it is commonly available as tinctures, gummies, and oils. Because of this lack of regulatory supervision, one research discovered that 26% of CBD products had less CBD than indicated, while 43% included much more. CBD appears to be relatively safe, with very minimal side effects such as sleepiness, diarrhea, and weight or hunger fluctuations. However, its safety for pregnant or nursing women is uncertain. CBD may interfere with drugs and have a negative influence on some health problems.

Cherry Juice with Tartness

Tart cherry juice, also known as sour cherry juice, appears to elevate melatonin levels and improve the availability of tryptophan, an amino acid that may aid with sleep. These are encouraging findings, because tart cherry juice may enhance sleep quality and make falling asleep simpler. Some research, however, suggest that the effect on insomnia is not as great as recognized therapies like as cognitive-behavioral therapy.

Tart cherries have been studied for their health advantages, with people consuming up to 270 cherries per day, but there has been no particular research into their safety. Before consuming the juice, which may be rather sour, it is normally diluted in a little amount of water.

Magnesium

Magnesium is a mineral that occurs naturally in food and is frequently added to processed meals. It is found in bones, soft tissue, and blood and is utilized throughout the body. Magnesium insufficiency is more common in older persons, and one of the mineral's numerous functions is sleep regulation. Some study shows that supplementary magnesium, either alone or in combination with melatonin and zinc, may help alleviate insomnia in older persons. It may also help people with excessive daytime drowsiness. Because large quantities of magnesium are found in foods such as pumpkin seeds, it is simple to supplement by eating more magnesium-rich foods. Magnesium supplements, including multivitamins, are also available in pill and tablet form. The magnesium aspartate, citrate, lactate, and chloride salts are the simplest for the body to absorb.

While magnesium is generally safe at normal dietary levels because the kidneys filter it out, large doses can induce diarrhea, nausea, and abdominal cramps. Magnesium also interacts with several medications and supplements, and high doses can cause serious heart problems such as low blood pressure or hypotension, irregular pulse, and cardiac arrest.

Gamma-aminobutyric acid (GABA)

Gamma-aminobutyric acid is a neurotransmitter and amino acid that regulates nervous system function. GABA is accessible as a supplement in addition to being produced by the body and found in foods like as tea and tomatoes. While it was originally thought that

GABA could not cross the blood-brain barrier and hence was useless to the body, there is now some evidence to the contrary.

Supplemental GABA has been found in small trials to lower tension and help people fall asleep more quickly. It is unclear if GABA's effects on sleep are related to stress reduction or another mechanism.

GABA exists naturally in the body and in food, but little study has been conducted to determine if it is safe to consume as a supplement. However, the majority of research have shown no negative effects. GABA comes in tablet form and can be obtained from natural or synthetic sources. The question of whether synthesized GABA is as effective as GABA produced from natural sources is still being researched.

Glycine

Glycine, like GABA, is an amino acid and neurotransmitter produced by the body and found in various foods. Glycine appears to have an effect on sleep and to cross the blood-brain barrier. Glycine appears to enhance sleep quality, possibly via reducing body temperature, according to research. Taking glycine before bedtime may also help lessen the impact of inadequate sleep on performance, which might be related to enhanced sleep quality or another reason.

Supplemental glycine is available in capsule or powder form, although it is unknown whether form is more useful. While glycine is included in our food, its safety in the proportions seen in supplements is uncertain.

Natural sleep aids

Natural sleep aids are not always harmless or dangerous. Natural sleep remedies are available over-the-counter or online.
Natural sleep aids are not always harmless or dangerous. Natural sleep aids, whether sold over-the-counter or online, do not go through the same testing and approval procedure as prescription medications.
There is a widespread dearth of high-quality research on the efficacy and safety of most natural sleep aids. As a result, many unanswered

issues concerning natural sleep therapies persist. When assessing the safety of natural sleep aids, there are a few things to bear in mind.

Adults

Many natural sleep cures have little negative effects when used in the recommended dosage by healthy individuals. However, this does not imply that all natural sleep aids are risk-free.

Adults should consult their doctor or pharmacist before using a natural sleep aid as a precaution. Adults should also discontinue using natural sleep aids if they experience any unusual health changes or negative effects.

Children

Some natural sleep aids may be safe for children to use, however sleep hygiene should be emphasized before using sleep aids. There is often inadequate evidence in children to properly assess the safety or efficacy of natural sleep aids.

Short-term use of certain natural sleep aids, such as melatonin, is usually regarded safe for most youngsters, but there is insufficient research on long-term usage.

To ensure that any medication or sleep aid does not negatively impact their child's health and development, parents should take the following precautions when considering natural sleep aids for their children:

Consulting their physician first; ensuring that the dose is appropriate for children rather than adults; paying attention to the label and ingredient list; and looking for high-quality goods that have been evaluated by third parties to decrease the danger of contaminated or mislabeled supplements.

People who are pregnant or breastfeeding

Natural sleep aids should be used with caution by pregnant or lactating women. Many substances have not been rigorously tested in pregnant or nursing women, so little is known about the possible consequences on their kid.

Although certain items may be safe, those who are pregnant or nursing should contact with their doctor before using natural sleep aids.

Before beginning to use any natural sleep aid, it is best to consult with a doctor. Despite the fact that these products are available without a prescription, your doctor may be able to assist you in numerous ways:

• Examining your other prescriptions and the possibility of interactions with a natural sleep aid.

• Discussing your medical history and the possibility of bad responses to natural sleep aids.

•Understanding your sleeping issues and determining whether they are the result of an underlying sleep disorder that may be treated with a more targeted approach.

• Examining the possible advantages and disadvantages of various natural sleep aids.
•providing dose or timing recommendations for natural sleep aids

•Explaining how to determine whether a natural sleep aid is effective or generating adverse effects.

Creating a sleep-friendly environment and developing healthy sleep habits are important for getting a good night's rest. Here are some tips to help you improve your sleep:

Make sure your bedroom is dark, cool, and quiet. Use heavy curtains or blinds to block out light, and use a fan or air conditioning to keep the room at a comfortable temperature. Also, use earplugs or a white noise machine to block out any outside noise.

Invest in a comfortable mattress and pillows. A supportive and comfortable sleeping surface can make a big difference in the quality of your sleep.

Establish a regular sleep schedule. Try to go to bed and wake up at the same time every day, even on weekends. This will help regulate your body's internal clock and make it easier to fall asleep and wake up.

Create a bedtime routine. Do the same things in the same order every night to signal to your body that it's time to sleep. This can include reading a book, listening to calming music, or taking a warm bath.

Avoid screens for at least an hour before bedtime. The blue light emitted by electronic devices can suppress the production of melatonin, making it harder to fall asleep.

Avoid caffeine, nicotine, and alcohol close to bedtime. These substances can all interfere with sleep, so it's best to avoid them for at least a few hours before going to bed.

Exercise regularly, but not close to bedtime. Regular physical activity can help you fall asleep faster and sleep more soundly, but it's best to avoid vigorous exercise close to bedtime, as it can make it harder to fall asleep.

Avoid heavy meals and big drinks close to bedtime. Eating a large meal close to bedtime can make it harder to fall asleep, as your body is busy digesting food. Similarly, drinking too much fluids before bed can cause you to wake up during the night to use the bathroom.

Keep your bedroom free of clutter. A messy and cluttered environment can be distracting and make it harder to fall asleep.

Avoid naps during the day. Napping during the day can disrupt your sleep schedule and make it harder to fall asleep at night.

By creating a sleep-friendly environment and developing healthy sleep habits, you can improve the quality of your sleep and feel more refreshed during the day. Remember, is not all about setting the perfect environment but also about incorporating healthy habits and lifestyle choices throughout the day that can contribute to a good night's rest.

CHAPTER 5

YOUR SKIN AND EMOTIONS ARE CONNECTED, even if you may not realize it. Consider how you feel when you are frightened, scared, or stressed. You may flush, sweat, or get hives. Glow skin is often connected with being in love. Stress can contribute to flares in those who have chronic skin diseases like psoriasis, eczema, or acne.

THE LINK BETWEEN THE SKIN AND THE EMOTIONS

To protect itself from infection and damage, the skin produces substances known as neuropeptides. They might induce inflammation, numbness, irritation, sensitivity, or tingling when released. The production of these chemicals during times of stress might aggravate pre-existing skin diseases such as psoriasis or eczema. Neuropeptides can also go to your brain, affecting the chemicals in your brain that help control emotions, leading to increased stress and, in turn, more skin issues.

Stress can also cause the skin's outer layer, or skin barrier function, to deteriorate, making it more sensitive and reactive. This may also indicate that your skin is more vulnerable to irritants, allergies, and germs.
Scientists believe it can aggravate rosacea, psoriasis, and dermatitis, make acne lesions more inflammatory and persistent, and produce hives or fever blisters.

Emotions, particularly negative emotions that can lead to anguish, worry, and despair, can influence not just the course of a disease but also the efficacy of therapy. According to Harvard Health, stress can interfere with your immune system, limiting your skin's ability to recover.

Psycho dermatology or psycho coetaneous medicine is the branch of medicine that studies the skin/mind link. In 1972, Stanford University established the first psycho dermatology clinic in the United States. Despite modest growth in this profession, there are already a number of clinics in the United States. The Association for

Psycho neurocutaneous Medicine of North America may help you identify a psycho dermatologist. When treating skin disorders, keep stress in mind.

There is no uniform response to stress. What is stressful to one person may be "no big problem" to another. And everyone of us may respond differently: some may get angry, some may be unable to sleep, while others may experience bodily symptoms such as nausea, migraines, tight muscles, or skin issues. According to Harvard Health, addressing both psychological causes and triggers of skin disorders may be beneficial for certain people. Stress reduction strategies are intended to make people feel more powerful and capable of dealing with daily challenges. They are most effective when used on a regular basis, as they reduce general feelings of stress. Many, however, can also be utilized in times of intense stress.

Mindfulness meditation, yoga, deep breathing, progressive muscle relaxation, exercise, listening to music, or indulging in a beloved activity are examples of relaxation techniques. Individual relaxation tactics may typically be mastered and incorporated into daily life. When done on a regular basis, many people report that their general stress levels reduce and that they are better equipped to handle challenging and stressful situations.

According to research, hypnosis, whether administered by a therapist or self-guided, can assist to reduce tension and anxiety, pain and inflammation, sweating and itching, hasten healing, and lessen harmful habits such as pulling hair, scratching lesions, or picking at sores.

Psychotherapy can be beneficial for certain people. Specific types of therapy, such as cognitive behavioral therapy, assist in replacing negative thought patterns that can increase stress or interfere with medical treatment with more realistic thoughts. Talking with a therapist about life's challenges might help reduce stress and improve skin conditions for some people. If you have a skin problem that is not responding to typical therapy, researching the skin/mind link, engaging with a therapist, or practicing stress reduction may be beneficial.

IMPORTANCE, BENEFITS, AND PRACTICES OF EMOTIONAL SELF-CARE

Self-care increases health and well-being and covers a variety of components. Emotional self-care is a component of self-care that many people ignore. Those who are easily agitated, upset, or burned out, whether in their dealings with people or in their employment, can use emotional self-care to enhance their emotional health and general quality of life.

Self-care is essentially taking care of oneself. It is taking time to rest or do activities that make us feel better physically, psychologically, and emotionally. Exercise, meditation, rest, spiritual activities, and treating oneself to regular bubble baths, spa days, or other gifts are examples of self-care acts. These activities can assist us in being healthier, reducing stress, and feeling better about ourselves.

Notably, in self-care, the individual is both the one acting and the one being acted upon, in contrast to other forms of care, such as dependent care, in which the person acting and the person being acted upon are distinct, and nursing care, in which the person acting acts on behalf of another (the patient, the patient's family, or hospital policy, for example).

Self-care, from a scientific standpoint, aims to "manage human functioning and human growth within standards consistent with life, health, and well-being."

The self-care process begins with studying and establishing one's self-care requirements, or whatever the individual requires to attain health and well-being norms. Then they must determine what to do to put these criteria into action, and ultimately, they must conduct acts or discontinue activity to achieve the intended result.

Someone who frequently feels fatigued throughout the day, for example, may explore and discover that they require more and/or better-quality sleep. They may then resolve to sleep early and avoid electronics for at least an hour before bed. The final stage would be to put the change into action. People frequently associate self-care activities with physical and mental well-being. However, the Substance Abuse and Mental Health Services Administration recommends that eight elements of self-care be addressed: physical, intellectual, spiritual, social, occupational, financial, environmental, and emotional.

Emotional self-care includes spending time recognizing and acknowledging your feelings, thoughts, and actions, as well as finding appropriate methods to express these emotions. It includes any acts you do to deal with stress, express emotions, and cultivate pleasant sentiments about life.

Many individuals believe they know their mood at any one time, yet unresolved emotions can have a significant influence on how they feel, their decisions, and their relationships with others. People commonly push bad feelings aside to be dealt with later or ignore them entirely because they do not want to linger on them. Those who do this may discover that they are not as fulfilled as they would want to be and may struggle to explain why.

WHY IS EMOTIONAL SELF-CARE IMPORTANT?

Taking care of your mental well-being enables you to feel better about yourself and more confident while dealing with unforeseen problems and relationship stumbling blocks. It may foster resilience and the ability to deal with change and the unavoidable hardships of life.

If someone does not properly care for their emotional health, they may suffer physical, mental, and social effects. They may become quickly overwhelmed, more upset when things do not go as planned, and unable of dealing with day-to-day issues. Kent University researchers discovered a link between emotions and health.

They discovered that people who linger on negative emotions are more likely to have physical and mental issues, whereas those who focus on the positive are healthier overall and live longer lives. Additional research indicates that people's bodies may suffer if their mental health is neglected. Long-term emotional conflict as a result of unpleasant or unresolved sentiments might exacerbate inflammation.

Long-term inflammation has been related to a variety of health problems, including cardiovascular disease, metabolic disorders, some forms of cancer, and brain and organ damage.

People who are going through a period of change might benefit from emotional self-care. For example, researchers at the University of Stirling in Scotland discovered in 2012 that persons with cancer benefit considerably from emotional self-care. A cancer diagnosis may cause a tremendous lot of upheaval in a person's life—their daily lives are disrupted by the treatment process, and their body and health undergo massive changes. The researchers discovered that emotional self-care measures assisted individuals in finding acceptance, reconstructing their identities, maintaining normality, and maintaining their sense of self.

THE ADVANTAGES OF EMOTIONAL SELF-CARE

Taking care of one's emotional well-being may enhance one's life in a variety of ways, in addition to improving one's physical health and lifespan. Resilience and balance have improved. Those who take care of their emotional health are more resilient, or capable of overcoming adversity and coping with the inherent obstacles of their lives and jobs.

Furthermore, emotional self-care can assist people in achieving internal and external life balance. Caring for one's health in all aspects develops equilibrium in the mind and body. Emotional self-care helps to manage duties and pressures such as job, family, and relationships, as well as one's personal needs. This is especially crucial for people who work in industries that frequently need a significant emotional involvement, such as the care professions.

IMPROVED SELF-ESTEEM

In a 2022 study, researchers from the Albert Einstein Hospital in So Paulo, Brazil, assessed stress, self-esteem, well-being, and cortisol levels in 120 health professionals who were randomly assigned to one of four groups, one of which was a control group with no intervention. Group participants completed questionnaires and had cortisol samples drawn before the intervention, 15 and 30 days later, and again during the 30-day follow-up. The intervention groups reported decreased stress, improved life satisfaction, higher self-esteem, and lower cortisol levels.
When someone can successfully identify, accept, and manage their emotions, their self-esteem rises. They may be able to recognize their desires more clearly when they build a life vision and purpose. This might motivate them to take additional constructive steps toward their own growth.

ENHANCED AUTHENTICITY

Emotional self-care is essentially rooted on self-compassion and understanding. It encourages authenticity by strengthening the connection to the human experience and increasing self-awareness. Those who adopt healthy ways of dealing with their emotions are better equipped to express themselves and behave in ways that are true to who they are and where they want to go in life.

RELATIONSHIPS THAT HAVE IMPROVED

Many people want emotional support from their spouses. Although this is a crucial function of partnerships, excessive dependence on one's spouse, or one partner relying on the other more than the other, can cause tension. When both partners practice emotional self-care, they stay in touch with and meet their own needs. When couples are able to maintain their sense of self-worth, satisfaction, and happiness apart from their relationship, they can come together and enjoy one another in a healthy, meaningful way without feeling pressed.

Furthermore, being aware of one's emotions leads to increased communication abilities, which enables for the formation of more significant and meaningful relationships with others.

DEPRESSION SYMPTOMS HAVE BEEN REDUCED

Emotional self-care can aid in the treatment of depression. At a 2022 study, researchers invited 800 cancer patients in an Iranian hospital to complete questionnaires to assess their depressive symptoms and self-care habits. The study found that high levels of emotional self-care, particularly self-efficacy practices, were related with decreased symptoms of depression.

EMOTIONAL SELF-CARE TECHNIQUES

Mindfulness and acceptance, healthy boundaries, positive self-talk, and relaxation are the four main components of practicing emotional self-care. The recommendations below will help you incorporate these habits into your life. Mindfulness and acceptance should be practiced.

Humans have a wide spectrum of emotions. It is critical to recognize that your sentiments are genuine and that there is no need to hide or reject them, and that self-judgment is neither helpful nor constructive. Self-acceptance practice allows you to be present, patient as you learn and grow, and accept all of your feelings. Expecting to feel just pleasant emotions all of the time is unrealistic; it is more useful to feel both positive and negative emotions as long as they are acknowledged and expressed in healthy ways.

SET AND KEEP HEALTHY BOUNDARIES

Prioritizing your needs and what is essential to you is part of emotional self-care. Saying no to things that aren't in your best interests or that may conflict with needed alone time is a sort of emotional self-care. It can be beneficial to spend some time to reflect on current limits as well as boundaries that need to be established, and to convey these when the circumstance calls for it. Once limits are established, it is critical to stick to them, even when it is unpleasant or inconvenient.

FIND PEACE

Taw-wab is a useful tool for establishing and enforcing boundaries in your life. Use Positive Self-Talk. We have no control over what people say about ourselves, but we can influence how we speak to and listen to ourselves. When faced with a challenging situation, we typically resort to self-criticism and humiliation. Learning to speak to oneself in healthy and good ways, just as you would to someone you love, is a crucial element of emotional self-care. Positive self-talk is linked to enhanced self-esteem, improved academic achievement, and athletic performance. Allow for Rest It is not good to perform at a high level all day; everyone requires pauses to unwind and recuperate. Allow yourself to pause when required. A break might take the shape of a nap or other state of relaxation, or it can consist of doing nothing for a few minutes. Taking a social media break can help you eliminate distractions, clear your mind, and focus on other tasks that demand your attention.

ADDITIONAL SUGGESTIONS

When it comes to emotional self-care, don't be afraid to think outside the box. There is no correct or incorrect strategy. The most essential thing is to develop a regimen that works for you—one person's emotional self-care may differ from another's. Here are a few more pointers to help you get started with emotional self-care in your everyday life:

• Incorporate emotional self-care into your everyday activities.

• Accept your wants and new experiences.

• Practice self- and other-forgiveness and appreciation.

• Begin journaling to express your ideas and emotions.

• Find a pastime and fun activities that allow you to express your creativity.

• Practice general self-care activities such as regular exercise, excellent sleep habits, meditation, and mindfulness.

• Work on self- and emotional management. Consider your actions and replies carefully; don't respond emotionally. Allow yourself to feel the feeling before deciding how to respond.

Above all, if you are having problems dealing with your emotions, get assistance. It is normal to feel exposed. Making a coffee date with a trusted friend, seeking advice from a family member, or organizing an appointment with a counselor or therapist might all be examples of this.

Maintaining emotional self-care does not imply always being or presenting happy. Emotional wellbeing entails accepting the good with the bad and embracing one's feelings for what they are. Those who exercise emotional self-care on a daily basis tend to control their emotions better and are more robust to change. Their relationships strengthen as a result of a stronger connection with others around them. Additionally, studies demonstrate that exercising emotional self-care might enhance physical health results.

Learning how to foster emotional intelligence and making time for things that create joy improves life quality. Take the time you need to understand, embrace, and control your emotions in healthy, productive ways.

Self-care has been professionally proved to lessen or eliminate anxiety and depression, stress, enhance focus, limit irritation and aggression, promote happiness, improve vitality, and more.

Have you ever observed that when you're anxious, your skin breaks out more? Perhaps your eczema or psoriasis has flared up, or your acne has become more difficult to manage? In any case, we've all seen how our bodies alter in reaction to stress, and your skin is not immune to that response!

For optimal health, many medical experts acknowledge that a natural balance between our sympathetic (fight-or-flight/high activity) and parasympathetic (rest-and-digest/relaxation) nerve systems must be maintained. Unfortunately, in today's environment, many of us suffer "Sympathetic Overdrive," which means that the time we spend in a state of high activity exceeds the time we spend in a condition of rest. This imbalance can cause a variety of health issues, such as insulin resistance (pre-diabetes), cardiovascular disease, and metabolic syndrome.
Increasing our time spent in the parasympathetic, or relaxed, state is an important aspect of reducing stress. While it is hard to escape stressful events in today's fast-paced society, we can change how we manage stress to prevent it from piling up.

See the list below for some ideas on how to include regular stress-reduction routines into your everyday life.

Prioritize Sleep

Many naturopathic physicians use the phrase "sleep hygiene" to promote a healthy sleep habit. Going to bed early and taking actions to encourage sleep in the evening, such as lowering the lights at a specific hour and avoiding food and drink after a certain time, are examples of sleep hygiene habits. Taking brief naps during the day can also help us improve our sleep hygiene and manage our stress levels.

Increase Your Physical Activity

Physical action helps to burn cortisol, a stress hormone, and strenuous exercise allows glucose to enter muscle cells without the need of insulin, which helps to control glucose and insulin activity. When beginning an exercise regimen, the most crucial factor to consider is if you love the activity enough to do it on a daily or weekly basis. To get your daily workout in, you don't need to go to the gym or sign up for a marathon; simply strolling around your neighborhood, watching internet fitness videos, or dancing around your house would enough. Learn more about selecting the best workout program for you here.

Try Mindfulness

Various mindfulness practices have been proved to be good for stress reduction and skin improvement. Yoga, meditation, tai chi, and deep breathing are some of these exercises. Check out this article on skin and mindfulness for additional information.

Improve Your Food Hygiene

Another phrase used by many naturopathic physicians, "food hygiene," relates to the environment in which we consume. Eating with people, eating without distractions, making and preparing your own food, chewing each mouthful thoroughly, paying attention to physical cues that suggest fullness, and avoiding multitasking while eating (i.e. no eating meals while watching TV!) are some techniques to enhance food hygiene.

Therapeutic Touch

Endorphins, which are released during physical touch, have been demonstrated in studies to significantly reduce stress. Getting a massage, offering more hugs, participating in more personal activities with your spouse, and playing with pets can all help us feel less stressed.

Eat a Balanced, Nutrient-Rich Diet

When we lack important nutrients, our bodies undergo metabolic stress. A whole food, plant-based diet rich in vegetables and fruits, healthy fats, and adequate protein, such as fish, nuts, and seeds, is the greatest method to satisfy our nutrient demands.

Do Things That Make You Pleasant

Because happiness stimulates endorphin production, you should laugh, dance, sing, join in community activities, garden, produce art, or engage in other happy hobbies to reduce stress.

Communicate with Someone

Interpersonal ties are essential for feeling supported and reducing stress. Participating in psychotherapy or simply conversing with family and friends can help reduce stress and create calm.

Connect with Nature

Shinrin-Yoku, which translates as "forest bathing," is a Japanese philosophy that promotes exposing oneself to nature for stress relaxation and illness prevention. This concept's advantages can be obtained by having home plants, going for walks outside, or trekking in a forest or park.

Try At-Home Therapeutics

To induce relaxation, try a warm herbal bath or foot bath, aromatherapy, an alternate shower (switch between hot and cold water), or other home-spa treatments, such as a DIY foot scrub or a self-massage with warming oils.

Reduce Toxins in Your Body

Drinking less alcohol, smoking less, and limiting other toxin-creating behaviors will help to reduce stress produced by the toxin burden on the body. It's also critical to understand which chemicals are present in your household and personal care items.

Consider Supplements

While supplements are not a replacement for a healthy diet, they can help compensate for vitamin deficiencies. Consider vitamin D3, B vitamins, and/or fish oil during the chilly winter months. Consult your doctor or a healthcare practitioner for more specific advice.

Drink Calming Herbal Teas

Many herbs are proven to promote relaxation and sleep. Lavender, chamomile, and peppermint, which has a cooling impact, are some relaxing herbal teas.

Meditation Has the Potential to Reduce Inflammation

Recent scientific research have shown that using Mindfulness-Based Stress Reduction (MBSR) practices on a regular basis can reduce inflammation. Psychological stress is a significant inflammatory trigger, and persons suffering from chronic inflammatory disorders frequently seek relief through stress reduction approaches.

WHAT IS THE PROCEDURE?

The brain responds to external stimuli, such as stressful events or trauma, by modifying and directing the immune system in order to properly respond. Another reaction implicated in the stress pathway is the production of cortisol, a hormone produced by the adrenal glands. One research evaluated the stress response and salivary cortisol levels after producing stress in experienced meditators go (over 6,000 lifetime hours of meditation) with non-meditators. The experienced meditators exhibited a statistically significant lower level of cortisol than the non-meditators.

A mindfulness-based movement program (including Yoga practice) was adopted in research participants for 8 weeks, with findings demonstrating a tendency toward reduced cortisol in those who exercised mindfulness-based movement compared to those who did not. There was also a substantial difference in other stress-related indicators.

One research revealed that yoga-based mindfulness practice lowered blood indicators of inflammation and stress, such as interleukin-6 (IL-6), tumor necrosis factor-alpha (TNF-a), and cortisol, in adults with chronic conditions within 10 days.

The relevance of IL-6 in skin inflammation is unknown, but this study provides another indication of yoga's therapeutic capacity to lower inflammatory markers. In a second investigation, 86 university employees were found to have elevated levels of an inflammatory blood marker known as "C-reactive protein." After two months of either Mindfulness-Based Stress Reduction (MBSR) or a general lifestyle education program, participants' inflammatory markers were assessed. Participants who practiced Mindfulness-Based Stress

Reduction (MBSR) had reduced CRP levels. Although CRP is a blood vessel inflammatory marker, it is not clear how it links to skin health.

SKIN INFLAMMATION CAUSED BY STRESS

The skin is one of the body's most visible lines of defense against invasion and damage, and the immune system protects against microbial infections. Furthermore, emotional and stress-related inflammation on the skin is extremely noticeable and can lead to inflammatory skin illnesses. The skin has several nerves that constitute a crucial network, which appears to be modularly by the brain. In fact, each square inch of skin contains 500+ nerve endings that link to the central nervous system! Psychological distress causes sensory nerves to release inflammatory molecules (for example, substance P), which combine with nor epinephrine (adrenaline) to cause inflammation in nearby immune cells and blood vessels. Many skin illnesses, including psoriasis, acne, atopic dermatitis, and alopecia, have been shown to worsen when stressed. Mindfulness-Based Stress Reduction (MBSR) might help with skin problems and general well-being.

Stress is an unavoidable part of life. Although some stress is acceptable and even necessary, excessive stress can have a negative impact on your quality of life and health. Simple actions may be done to assist reduce tension.

Stress-Relieving Techniques

• Take calm, deep breaths when you are agitated.

• Take a warm bath.

• Play relaxing music.

• Go for a stroll or engage in another activity.

• Pray or meditate.

• Attend a yoga class.

• Get a massage or a back rub.

• Drink something warm that doesn't include alcohol or caffeine.

You may also make some modifications to your daily behaviors to lessen and relieve stress

• Get plenty of rest.

• Maintain contact with family, friends, and other caring individuals in your life.

• Engage in regular physical activity.

It can assist you in clearing your thoughts and releasing feelings of irritation and worry.

• Avoid caffeine-containing beverages and foods. Caffeine might make you feel tense and agitated.

• Avoid smoking and using tobacco.

• Avoid consuming alcohol. It can induce insomnia and despair.

Muscle relaxation to ease stress

When you are stressed, your body may stiffen up, which can produce discomfort. Muscle tension and anxiety can be reduced if you learn to relax your muscles. Progressive muscular relaxation is an activity that can help you with this.

In progressive muscle relaxation, you contract and then relax linked muscle groups. You might use a relaxation tape or CD to assist you go through all of the muscle groups. You may also memorize the muscle groups and practice through them from memory.

Find a peaceful location where you will not be harassed. Check that you can comfortably lie on your back.

For each muscle group, do the following:

Take a deep breath and tighten the muscle group for 4 to 10 seconds.
Tense up, but not so much that you cramp.
Exhale while abruptly and totally relaxing the muscle group. Don't let it go gradually.
Take a 10- to 20-second break.

Arms and hands

Make a tight fist with your hands.
Tense your wrists and forearms and bend your hands back at the wrist.
Biceps and upper arms: Form fists with your hands, bend your arms at the elbows, and tighten your biceps.
Shrug your shoulders.

The head and neck

• Make a deep frown on your forehead.

• Close your eyelids as firmly as possible around the eyes and bridge of the nose. Remove your contact lenses before commencing the workout.

• Cheeks and jaws: Make the widest possible smile.

• Close your lips tightly around your mouth.

• Neck: Push your head back against the floor or chair.

• Front of the neck: Place your chin against your chest.

The upper body

• Chest: Take a deep breath, hold it, and then exhale.

• Back: Arch your back up and away from the chair or the floor.

• Stomach: Squeeze it tightly.

The lower body

• Hips and back end (buttocks): Tightly squeeze the buttocks together.

• Thighs: Squeeze them tightly.

• Lower legs: Extend your heels and flex your toes up, as if you were attempting to bring your toes up to touch your shins. Then curl your toes downward and point them away.

This workout may cause you to feel drowsy. Count backwards from 5 to 1 to "wake up" your body. Then make movements with your fingers, toes, hands, and feet. Finally, move and stretch your entire body.

Before you drive or engage in other activities, be sure you are aware. Roll breathing improves lung function and puts you in touch with your breathing pattern. You may do it in any posture, but lying on your back with your legs bent is the best. Roll breathing should be practiced regularly for many weeks until you can perform it practically anywhere.

Always breathe in through your nose and out through your mouth during rolling breathing. Make a whooshing sound as you exhale.

Put your left hand on your stomach and your right hand on your chest. Take note of how your hands move as you inhale and exhale.

Inhale deeply to fill your lower lungs. As you do this, your tummy will push your left hand up. Your right hand is frozen. After that, exhale. As your tummy sinks, so will your left hand. Repeat 8 to 10 times.

Continue to breathe in as previously, but don't stop when your left hand pushes up. Continue to inhale. You should feel your upper chest expand and your right hand rise. As your tummy sinks, so will your left hand.

Exhale slowly via your mouth. Feel the stress leave your body as you exhale. Both of your hands will drop.

Repeat for 3 to 5 minutes. Take note of how your tummy and chest move like waves, rising and falling steadily.

Take note of how you feel after you breathe in this manner.

SUMMARY

REDUCED RISK OF CHRONIC DISEASES

Regular physical activity and exercise, abalanced diet, and maintaining a healthy weight can lower the risk of chronic diseases such as heart disease, diabetes, and certain cancers.

Improved mood and cognitive function

Eating a healthy diet that includes fruits, vegetables, whole grains, and lean proteins can provide the nutrients that the brain needs to function properly. Regular physical activity can also help to reduce stress, anxiety, and depression.

Increased energy levels

Regular physical activity and eating a balanced diet can help to increase energy levels, allowing individuals to accomplish more throughout the day.

Improved sleep

Regular physical activity, avoiding caffeine and heavy meals before bed, and maintaining a consistent sleep schedule can help to improve sleep quality.

Enhanced immune function

Regular physical activity, a balanced diet, and adequate sleep can all help to enhance the immune system and reduce the risk of illness.

BETTER PHYSICAL APPEARANCE

A healthy lifestyle can help people to achieve and maintain a healthy weight, toned muscles, and a clear complexion.

Improved self-esteem and self-confidence

Achieving and maintaining a healthy weight and a healthy overall appearance can help to improve self-esteem and self-confidence.

Increased lifespan

Adopting a healthy lifestyle can help people to live a longer, healthier life.

Better overall quality of life

Maintaining a healthy lifestyle can help to improve overall physical and mental well-being, leading to a better overall quality of life.

It's worth noting that The benefits of maintaining a healthy lifestyle go beyond just physical health. The mental and emotional benefits of a healthy lifestyle can be just as important, if not more so. It can be challenging to make lifestyle changes, but the rewards of doing so are well worth the effort and commitment.

All in all, a healthy lifestyle is a lifestyle that brings physical, mental and emotional benefits, it is a lifetime commitment and the effort and dedication to achieve it will lead to a better quality of life, longer lifespan, improved self-esteem and self-confidence, in addition to reducing the risk of chronic diseases.

www.ingramcontent.com/pod-product-compliance
Lightning Source LLC
Chambersburg PA
CBHW071042250726
48653CB00005B/1950